ORYX SCIENCE BIBLIOGRAPHIES

Volume 7

AIDS

(Acquired Immune Deficiency Syndrome)

Second Edition

by David A. Tyckoson

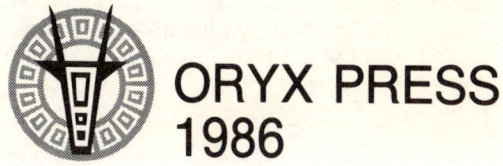

ORYX PRESS
1986

The rare Arabian Oryx is believed to have inspired the myth of the unicorn. This desert antelope became virtually extinct in the early 1960s. At that time several groups of international conservationists arranged to have 9 animals sent to the Phoenix Zoo to be the nucleus of a captive breeding herd. Today the Oryx population is over 400, and herds have been returned to reserves in Israel, Jordan, and Oman.

Copyright © 1986 by David A. Tyckoson

Published by The Oryx Press
2214 North Central at Encanto
Phoenix, AZ 85004-1483

Published simultaneously in Canada

All rights reserved
No part of this publication may be reproduced or transmitted in any form or by any means, electronic or mechanical, including photocopying, recording, or by any information storage and retrieval system, without permission in writing from The Oryx Press.

Printed and Bound in the United States of America

Library of Congress Cataloging-in-Publication Data

Tyckoson, David A.
  AIDS (Acquired immune deficiency syndrome)

  (Oryx science bibliographies ; v. 7)
  Includes index.
  1. AIDS (Disease)—Bibliography. 2. AIDS (Disease)—Abstracts. I. Title. II Series. [DNLM: 1. Acquired Immunodeficiency Syndrome—abstracts. ZWD 308 T978a]
Z6664.A27T9   1986   016.61697'92   86-42747
[RC607.A26]
ISBN 0-89774-323-7

Table of Contents

About the Series	1
Research Review: Update on AIDS	3
Medical Aspects of AIDS	11
Epidemiology and Transmission	17
AIDS, the Blood Supply, and the AIDS Blood Test	24
AIDS and Intravenous Drug Users	33
AIDS Outside of the High Risk Groups	34
The Search for an AIDS Cure	38
AIDS Hysteria, Fears, and Fallacies	46
Case Studies of AIDS Victims	53
AIDS and Health Care Workers	55
AIDS in Prisons, the Military, and the Workplace	57
Psychological Aspects of AIDS	61
Changes in Sexual Behavior Due to AIDS	64
The Legal Problems of AIDS	67
AIDS and the Schools	68
AIDS and the Church	70
AIDS Research, Funding, and Economic Impact	71
The Patent Rights to the AIDS Virus	74
Services for AIDS Victims	78
Rock Hudson: AIDS Strikes a Star	80
AIDS Outside the United States	82
Animal AIDS	86
Author Index	87

About the Series

The <u>Oryx Science Bibliographies</u> are a new series of bibliographies designed to bring you the most recent references on the current issues in the sciences. Each issue will provide between 200-400 fully annotated references along with a "Research Review" covering the history and state of the art of the topic being covered. These bibliographies are intended to provide the student or researcher with an effective introduction to the hot topics in the sciences. Each bibliography contains a number of special features, such as:

Evaluative Selection: The bibliographer reviews each article to ensure that only the most valuable references are included. The bibliography does not strive to be comprehensive but to include only the most important items on the topic.

Fully Annotated: All of the references are annotated, providing a useful summary of the source materials for the user.

Readily Available Materials: All references chosen for inclusion are available at most libraries throughout the United States and Canada. Obscure sources that are difficult to obtain are usually avoided.

Highly Current: The bibliography strives to include the most recent materials to keep it as up to date as possible. References from as recently as the last six months before publication may be found in all issues.

Key Articles Highlighted: The most important articles in each bibliography are highlighted in **boldface** so that the user interested in only a few references can key in to those that are the most useful.

Research Review: Each issue contains a research review describing the state of the art of the subject being covered.

Undergraduate Level: Only materials that are written at the undergraduate student level are chosen. Neither highly technical nor extremely general articles are included.

English Language Only: Only English language materials are included.

Research Review: Update on AIDS

Since the publication of the first AIDS bibliography in the Oryx Science Bibliographies series in January 1985, much new information has been discovered about the disease and it has become much more embedded in the American consciousness. More literature appeared during 1985 and the first half of 1986 than was written throughout the entire previous history of AIDS. This bibliography reflects that influx of AIDS into the scientific and popular literature in that it contains almost twice as many references as the first edition. All of the sources abstracted in this volume have either been published since the first volume was published or were otherwise excluded in that bibliography. No references are repeated from the first edition.

Medical Aspects of AIDS

The medical conditions known as the Acquired Immune Deficiency Syndrome have not changed appreciably since the disease was first described and studied. It is caused by a virus, alternately known as the Human T-cell Leukemia Virus Type III (HTLV-III), the Lymphadenopathy Associated Virus (LAV), or the Human Immunodeficiency Virus (HIV), that attacks the immune system and leaves the body open to secondary infections. These infections, most commonly Kaposi's sarcoma or pneumocystis carinii pneumonia, overcome the victim and eventually lead to the death of the patient. The virus is highly infectious but not very contagious and there is an extremely long lead time (often many years) from exposure to contracting the disease, which complicates the identification and study of AIDS. Over 16,000 cases of AIDS have already been confirmed and 12,000 new cases are expected in 1986. No one has ever recovered completely from AIDS and there is still no known cure or vaccine.

While most cases of AIDS worldwide are found in the United States, many other nations are also experiencing an AIDS crisis. Hundreds of cases have been reported in Europe and the Caribbean and sporadic cases have been found in the middle east, the Indian subcontinent, the far east, and the Soviet Union. Many scientists theorize that the virus originated in central Africa, but the governments of nations in that region do not admit that AIDS is a problem. African scientists view this theory as another slur against the continent of Africa and feel that Africa is blamed for every new problem afflicting the western world.

High Risk Groups

AIDS is most frequently associated with four high risk groups: male homosexuals (73% of all victims), intravenous drug users (17%), blood transfusion recipients (3%), and female sexual partners of male AIDS victims (1%). Haitian immigrants, who were initially included as another high risk group, have recently been removed from that category.

Six percent of all cases involve patients who do not fit into any of these classifications.

AIDS Outside of the High Risk Groups

The largest percentage increase in AIDS cases has occurred in those people outside of the high risk groups, particularly women and children. Increasing evidence indicates that the virus can be sexually transmitted from men to women and possibly from women to men. In order to avoid contracting AIDS, both women and men need to become more selective in their sexual practices. Children are the most unfortunate of AIDS victims, with hundreds of confirmed cases having been reported in children under thirteen years of age. Most of these victims were exposed to the virus before birth or contracted AIDS through blood transfusions. Women who have been exposed to the AIDS virus should carefully consider risking a pregnancy and passing the disease on to their children.

Transmission of the AIDS Virus

There are only three ways to transmit the AIDS virus from one person to another: injection of the virus into the bloodstream, sexual contact with an AIDS victim, or mother to child during pregnancy. Sexual transmission is the most common method of transmission and certain sexual practices are considered to be more dangerous than others. Anal and oral sex allow the virus an easier pathway into the bloodstream than heterosexual intercourse. The virus has been isolated from other bodily secretions of AIDS patients, particularly saliva and tears, but there is absolutely no evidence that the virus can be transmitted in this form. Without access to the bloodstream, the virus cannot infect another individual. Casual contact with an AIDS victim poses no health hazard.

The AIDS Blood Test

One of the biggest advances of the last two years has been the development and commercial use of a blood test for exposure to the AIDS virus. The test most commonly in use is the enzyme-linked immunosorbent assay (ELISA), which detects antibodies to the AIDS virus but not the virus itself. This test is easy and inexpensive to run, but it produces a high number of false positive readings. These false positive results may indicate that a person has been exposed to the virus when in fact they have not. Any positive samples must be tested a second time using the more expensive but more accurate Western Blot or Immunofluorescence tests. The primary use of the ELISA blood test is to screen blood donations at blood banks to prevent the spread of AIDS through transfusions. It has apparently been successful in this goal because the number of cases of hemophiliacs who have AIDS has stabilized and is even decreasing.

Patent Rights to the AIDS Virus

The ELISA blood test represented the first mass commercial application of any AIDS research and brought with it an instant business market worth millions of dollars. Because of the obvious potential for royalties related to this and future AIDS-related tests, vaccines, and cures, a priority fight is currently underway on the patent rights to the AIDS virus. The virus was originally discovered by a French research team and named the LAV virus. Shortly after this, an American group headed by Dr. Robert Gallo announced that HTLV-III was the AIDS virus. This report received a great deal more publicity and since then Dr. Gallo has usually been given credit for the discovery of the virus. He filed for and received a patent in the United States for the HTLV-III virus, despite the fact that the French group had filed first. The French team is now suing the National Institutes of Health for infringement. To complicate matters further, a correction to Dr. Gallo's original paper identifying the AIDS virus notes that the electron micrograph accompanying the article was really a picture of the LAV virus and not the HTLV-III as indicated. While not entirely resolved at this time, this admission of error, along with a Patent Office ruling favoring the French claim, seems to indicate that the French research team is the true discoverer of the AIDS virus and should receive any royalty payments resulting from that discovery.

As the patent fight rages on, an international team of experts has been convened to give an official name to the virus. In a compromise to both LAV and HTLV-III, this team has proposed the use of Human Immunodeficiency Virus (HIV) as the official name. While the NIH French team is willing to agree to this nomenclature, Dr. Gallo and the NIH still intend to use HTLV-III. Until this matter is resolved, the AIDS virus will have at least two and possibly three different names. This infighting will also undoubtably slow down the research on finding a cure for AIDS until the matter is resolved.

The Search for a Cure

Ever since the AIDS virus was first identified, scientists have been trying to discover a method to protect the body from its effects and to stop the virus from spreading. The most important development so far has been the identification of the complete genome sequence of the AIDS virus. Knowing this genetic code, it may be possible for researchers to genetically engineer an inactive virus that can be used to create an AIDS vaccine. Work is currently underway on this project, but a commercially available vaccine will probably not be available for at least four more years.

While some scientists are looking for an AIDS vaccine, others are searching for drugs that can either strengthen a patient's immune system or stop the secondary infections that lead to the death of the victim. Many different drugs have been tested, but none has yet been shown to be completely effective. Isoprinosine, suramin, ribavirin, cyclosporine, azidothymidine, and HPA-23 have been the most commonly used drugs, but most of these are not approved by the FDA for use in the United States. One unfortunate sidelight of the AIDS crisis is that some unscrupulous individuals are selling ineffective cures and false hopes to desperate victims in order to profit from their disease.

Psychological Aspects of AIDS

AIDS victims suffer not only from the physical aspects of their disease but from psychological factors as well. Many AIDS patients are shunned by their family and friends, left to die a slow painful death in isolation. This leads to severe depression and other mental disorders. Physicians and health care personnel must consider the mental as well as the physical well being of the patients with whom they work. There is also evidence that the AIDS virus attacks the brain and directly causes some of the neurological disorders in its victims. These symptoms have been labeled AIDS dementia and are becoming more widespread among AIDS victims.

Health Care Workers and AIDS

The only occupational group that is at any direct risk for AIDS is the health care community. Although AIDS cannot be transmitted through casual contact, health care workers must be careful when handling blood samples and bodily fluids from AIDS patients. Two possible cases of AIDS transmission in the hospital have occurred, one involving a nurse with needlestick injuries and another involving the accidental injection of blood from an AIDS patient into a nurse. Although this is only a minute percentage of the many thousands of hospital and health care employees dealing with AIDS victims on a daily basis, the Centers for Disease Control have issued guidelines to protect the safety of these workers.

Ethical and Legal Problems of AIDS

Because the AIDS blood test only indicates if a person has antibodies to the virus and not the virus itself, this test cannot be used as a predictor to identify who will eventually contract AIDS. This has resulted in a number of ethical and legal problems related to the use of the test. If an individual has a positive result on an AIDS test, does that person have the right to know the test results? Should all positive results be reported to the government or other institutions? The confidentiality of medical test results must be balanced against the public health concerns of the state in its efforts to halt the spread of the disease. When these two priorities conflict, there are no clear answers to the dilemma.

Several lawsuits have already appeared over the accidental spread of the AIDS virus. A few individuals who contracted AIDS through the blood supply have brought suits against the blood banks and physicians responsible for their treatment. One nurse has sued her hospital for failure to notify her that she was treating an AIDS patient and even Rock Hudson's lover is suing the Hudson estate on the basis that Mr. Hudson did not inform his sexual partner that he had AIDS. The number of AIDS cases in the courts will probably increase dramatically over the next few years and could become a legal nightmare.

In order to prevent such lawsuits, some businesses and other institutions would like to use the blood test to screen all new and/or current employees in order to keep out AIDS victims and to prevent the transmission of AIDS in the workplace. Despite the fact that AIDS cannot be transmitted through casual contact, the United States military has begun a program to screen all new recruits, insurance companies are issuing AIDS blood tests to members of all high risk groups who apply for new policies, and the Justice Department has approved the firing of anyone who tests positive for antibodies to the AIDS virus. Gay rights groups believe that this is only a thinly veiled mask to keep homosexuals out of the military and the business community.

Not all of the news about AIDS has been bad. Many social service agencies have established support groups, hospices, and educational programs for AIDS victims, their friends, and their families. Through the experiences of services such as the Gay Men's Health Crisis in New York City and the Shanti Project in San Francisco, AIDS victims have found sources of information and support. Some churches have also helped AIDS patients, following the example of Jesus in ministering to the sick and dispossessed. The experiences of these initial service organizations should break the ground for other such services to become established.

AIDS Hysteria

Fear of AIDS is even more pervasive and potentially more dangerous than the disease itself. Because there is no known cure and no one has ever recovered, AIDS has become the most publicized and least understood disease of our time. Due to either uncertainty or unwillingness to report detailed sexual material, the news media has not been explicit enough in telling the public how the AIDS virus can be transmitted. This lack of knowledge has caused much of the public to shun AIDS victims out of fear of contracting the disease. Some parents have even kept their children out of school if the child was in the same classroom as an AIDS victim. Others have advocated the isolation of all AIDS victims so that they may have no other contacts with society. These ideas are all based on the mistaken notion that AIDS can be transmitted through everyday exposure to a victim.

The public's lack of knowledge about the disease is also being used in a more sinister way by those who want to discriminate against members of the high risk groups, particularly homosexuals and drug users. Some fundamentalist religious leaders are claiming that AIDS is retribution for sins against God and that all AIDS victims deserve their fates. Others are using AIDS to keep homosexuals out of the workforce, the military, and other institutions that have traditionally been intolerant of gays. While the AIDS blood test only identifies the presence of antibodies to the AIDS virus and does not indicate if any one individual has AIDS or how it was transmitted, some institutions and individuals are viewing a positive result on the blood test as an admission of either intravenous drug use or homosexuality. Proper education is needed so that the public can become fully aware of the facts and the fiction surrounding AIDS.

Sexual Behavior Changes Due to AIDS

Because of this fear of AIDS, the sexual revolution may be coming to an end. Since sexual promiscuity increases the chances of catching the disease, many men and women have greatly decreased their number of sexual contacts. Sex with a large number of unknown partners is becoming a much more rare activity among both homosexuals and heterosexuals. Many individuals are engaging in long term monogamous relationships or are having sex only with known partners. The methods used in sexual experiences are also changing. Because anal and oral sex are the most likely methods of spreading the virus, many individuals are only using other sexual methods, are only having sex while wearing condoms, or both.

Rock Hudson: AIDS Strikes a Star

The public became fully aware of the pervasiveness of AIDS when it became known that one of the film industry's biggest stars had the disease, Rock Hudson. Mr. Hudson, who had always led a very private life off screen, instantly became the most famous AIDS victim in the world. This was not publicity that he desired, but his illness did more to raise the consciousness of the American public than any other single AIDS patient. Because a celebrity now had AIDS, donations for AIDS research began coming in from people in the film industry and other concerned individuals across the nation. When Mr. Hudson announced that he had AIDS, he was on his way to Paris to try the experimental drug HPA-23. Unfortunately, this drug had no effect on his condition and he passed away a short time later.

The Future of AIDS

The prospects for eliminating AIDS as a health threat do not look any better than they did two years ago. Researchers have now identified the genetic sequence of the virus, but a vaccine still appears to be at least four years away. Some experimental drugs are being used to combat the virus and the secondary infections, but none has yet been very successful. The AIDS blood test can identify who has been exposed to the virus, but it cannot predict who will eventually get the disease. Because of the very long lead time between exposure and infection, scientists cannot even predict how many AIDS cases will be confirmed in the future. The virus is spreading far beyond the initial high risk groups and is a threat to anyone participating in sexual activity or receiving blood transfusions. In addition to the health threat, fear of the disease is being used to overtly discriminate against members of the high risk groups. While scientists search for a cure or a vaccine, the media must educate the public on the real and imaginary threats of AIDS. Only public education and diligent medical research can help to stop the AIDS crisis. It is hoped that this bibliography will help by providing the public with an index to informative materials about AIDS from all medical and political perspectives.

David A. Tyckoson
Iowa State University
July 1986

Medical Aspects of AIDS

1. Abrams, Donald I. "Lymphodenopathy Related to the Acquired Immunodeficiency Syndrome in Homosexual Men." Medical Clinics of North America, v. 70, May 1986, pp. 693-706.
    Persistent generalized lymphodenopathy is commonly associated with AIDS. Clinical and laboratory findings may be able to predict which patients will progress from this condition to full-blown AIDS.

2. "Acquired Immunodeficiency Syndrome: Meeting of the WHO Collaborating Centers on AIDS." MMWR: Morbidity and Mortality Weekly Report, v. 34, November 8, 1985, pp. 678-679.
    The World Health Organization has established a network of collaborating centers to facilitate international cooperation on AIDS research. The CDC definition of AIDS was approved as the WHO definition and a series of guidelines for AIDS researchers were developed and are summarized in this report.

3. "AIDS Update." Science News, v. 128, July 20, 1985, p. 40.
    Recent AIDS research indicates that the virus operates by disabling the T-4 cells, which are the white blood cells that recognize and respond to foreign proteins. Antibodies taken from the blood of AIDS patients may be somewhat effective in preventing the disease. Several other symptoms have recently been added to the list of AIDS indicators.

4. "AIDS Update (Part I)." Harvard Medical School Health Letter, v. 10, November 1985, pp. 1-4.
    AIDS is caused by the HTLV-III virus, which results in a destruction of the immune system and has no known cure. At present researchers are looking for a method to treat the secondary infections and ultimately to develop a vaccine to the virus itself.

5. Allan, J. S. et al. "Major Glycoprotein Antigens That Induce Antibodies in AIDS Patients Are Encoded by HTLV-III." Science, v. 228, May 31, 1985, pp. 1091-1094.
    Antibodies from the serum of patients with AIDS recognize two major glycoproteins in cells infected with HTLV-III. It is hypothesized that these two glycoproteins are directly involved in the pathology of HTLV-III infection.

6. Barin, F. et al. "Virus Envelope Protein of HTLV-III Represents Major Target Antigen for Antibodies in AIDS Patients." Science, v. 228, May 31, 1985, pp. 1094-1096.
    Two glycoproteins encoded by HTLV-III were the most consistently recognized by antibodies to the virus. The ability to detect these areas may be valuable in establishing the presence or absence of antibodies to the virus.

7. Barre-Sinoussi, Francoise et al. "Isolation of Lymphadenopathy-Associated Virus (LAV) and Detection of LAV Antibodies from U.S. Patients with AIDS." <u>JAMA: Journal of the American Medical Association</u>, v. 253, March 22, 1985, pp. 1737-1739.

A retrovirus was isolated from the blood of AIDS patients and shown to be identical to the LAV virus. This supports the theory that LAV causes AIDS.

8. Baum, Rudy. "AIDS Virus Genome Sequenced." <u>Chemical and Engineering News</u>, v. 63, February 18, 1985, pp. 32-34.

Three research groups have all reported independently that they have found the complete nucleotide sequence of the AIDS virus. Now that the genetic makeup of the virus is known, it may be possible to find a vaccine or cure for the disease.

9. Burkes, Ronald L. et al. "Simultaneous Occurrence of Pneumocystis Carinii Pneumonia, Cytomegalovirus Infection, Kaposi's Sarcoma, and B-Immunoblastic Sarcoma in a Homosexual Man." <u>JAMA: Journal of the American Medical Association</u>, v. 253, June 21, 1985, pp. 3425-3428.

A case study of a man with AIDS who contracted Pneumocystis carinii, cytomegalovirus infection, Kaposi's sarcoma, and B-cell immunoblastic sarcoma simultaneously. A compromised immune system led to these infections and resultant death.

10. "Cofactor in AIDS?" <u>Science News</u>, v. 128, August 3, 1985, p. 77.

Cytomegalovirus may be a hidden cofactor in the development of AIDS. A study of men who have been exposed to the AIDS virus but who have not yet contracted AIDS reveals that one-half have also been infected by cytomegalovirus.

11. "Diarrhea and Malabsorbtion Associated with the Acquired Immunodeficiency Syndrome (AIDS)." <u>Nutrition Reviews</u>, v. 43, August 1985, pp. 235-237.

AIDS patients frequently exhibit unexplained diarrhea, malabsorption, and weight loss. Any patients who show these signs and are at risk for the disease should be evaluated for AIDS.

12. Gottlieb, Michael S. "Immunologic Aspects of the Acquired Immunodeficiency Syndrome and Male Homosexuality." <u>Medical Clinics of North America</u>, v. 70, May 1986, pp. 651-664.

A review of the immunologic aspects of AIDS and AIDS-related syndromes, including etiology and pathogenesis. Predisposing factors for AIDS in both homosexual and bisexual men are presented.

13. "Intracranial Lesions in AIDS." *American Family Physician*, v. 32, September 1985, pp. 206-209.

Of thirty-three AIDS patients with neurologic problems who had CAT scans, twenty-seven demonstrated abnormalities. The appearance of lesions in the brain may be sufficient evidence for a diagnosis of toxoplasmosis in AIDS patients.

14. "Isobutyl Nitrite and AIDS." *American Family Physician*, v. 32, November 1985, p. 272.

The inhalation of isobutyl nitrite may damage the immune system and increase the risk of AIDS. This drug is often used as an aphrodisiac by homosexual men.

15. Johnstone, Bob. "Does Prostaglandin Aid the AIDS Virus?" *New Scientist*, v. 110, April 10, 1986, p. 28.

Prostaglandin E2 may assist in the transmission of AIDS among homosexual men. This hormone-like compound is present in large amounts in semen and is easily absorbed into the blood stream.

16. Kenton, Charlotte. "Acquired Immunodeficiency Syndrome (AIDS)." *National Library of Medicine Literature Search*, **issued quarterly by the National Library of Medicine, April 1983 - present. Superintendent of Documents Number HE20.3614/2:**

A quarterly bibliography of world-wide medical research on AIDS.

17. Kristal, Alan R. "The Impact of the Acquired Immunodeficiency Syndrome on Patterns of Premature Death in New York City." *JAMA: Journal of the American Medical Association*, v. 255, May 2, 1986, pp. 2306-2310.

The AIDS mortality rate in 1984 for persons aged 15 to 64 was 42.2 per 100,000 for males and 5.3 for females. AIDS is the leading cause of death for males aged 30 to 39 and is among the top five causes for all males. AIDS has had a significant effect on the premature mortality rate.

18. Langone, John. "AIDS: Special Report." *Discover***, v. 6, December 1985, pp. 28-53.**

AIDS is a terrible disease that destroys the immune system and leaves the body open to secondary infections. No one has yet recovered from the disease and one half of all victims have died. The methods of transmission and infection are described.

19. Laurence, Jeffrey. "The Immune System in AIDS." *Scientific American*, v. 253, December 1985, pp. 84-93.

The AIDS virus infects the T-4 cells and alters their growth. These cells are slowly eliminated and the immune system fails to function properly. The search is on for an antiviral drug to use as a vaccine against AIDS.

20. Marwick, Charles. "Molecular Level View Gives Immune System Clues." <u>JAMA: Journal of the American Medical Association</u>, v. 253, June 21, 1985, pp. 3371-3376.

The HTLV-III virus works by destroying the T-4 cells which produce antibodies. The exact mechanisms of the virus are explained.

21. Mason, James O. "Public Health Service Plan for the Prevention and Control of Acquired Immune Deficiency Syndrome (AIDS)." <u>Public Health Reports</u>, **v. 100, September/October 1985, pp. 453-455.**

The Public Health Service has determined the key goals and objectives that must be met to achieve the prevention and control of AIDS. Specific problems, assumptions, goals, and objectives in fighting the disease are presented.

22. Muggia, Franco M. and Mathew Lonberg. "Kaposi's Sarcoma and AIDS." <u>Medical Clinics of North America</u>, v. 70, January 1986, pp. 139-154.

The underlying factor in AIDS is a profound defect in the immune system. This often allows the otherwise rare form of cancer known as Kaposi's sarcoma to develop. A review of Kaposi's sarcoma associated with AIDS is presented.

23. O'Sullivan, Peggy, Ruth A. Linke, and Sharron Dalton. "Evaluation of Body Weight and Nutritional Status Among AIDS Patients." <u>Journal of the American Dietetic Association</u>, v. 85, November 1985, pp. 1483-1484.

A large proportion of AIDS patients are at nutritional risk. Most victims suffer a large weight loss associated with AIDS. Proper nutrition may help to slow the effects of the disease.

24. "Pneumonia in AIDS Patients." <u>American Family Physician</u>, v. 33, January 1986, p. 266.

Pneumocystis carinii is the organism most responsible for AIDS-related pneumonia. Methods for identifying this condition are given and some other causes of AIDS-related pneumonia are explored.

25. "Pulmonary Complications of AIDS." <u>American Family Physician</u>, v. 31, March 1985, p. 215.

Of fifty-two patients with pulmonary complications related to AIDS, thirty-four showed normal or near normal chest x-rays. Doctors should be aware that a normal x-ray does not mean that no infection has occurred.

26. Quinn, Thomas C. "Perspectives On the Future of AIDS." <u>JAMA: Journal of the American Medical Association</u>, v. 253, January 11, 1985, pp. 247-249.

As the AIDS crisis spread, medical researchers quickly identified the HTLV-III virus as the cause. A new test has just been developed to examine blood for antibodies to AIDS. We will now have the capability to study the further spread of the disease.

27. "Radiotherapy for AIDS-Related Kaposi's Sarcoma." American Family Physician, v. 31, April 1985, pp. 245-246.

Kaposi's sarcoma in AIDS patients differs from that of non-AIDS sufferers in that it may occur anywhere on the body. Radiation therapy may be successful in controlling AIDS-related Kaposi's sarcoma.

28. Ratner, L. et al. "Complete Nucleotide Sequence of the AIDS Virus, HTLV-III." Nature, v. 313, January 1986, pp. 277-280.

The complete gene sequence of the HTLV-III virus is presented.

29. "Revision of the Case Definition of Acquired Immunodeficiency Syndrome for National Reporting: United States." MMWR: Morbidity and Mortality Weekly Reports, v. 34, June 28, 1985, pp. 373-375.

Since the definition of AIDS was developed in 1982, the HTLV-III/LAV virus has been found to be the causative factor in the disease. The definition has been revised to take into account this and other developments in the study of AIDS.

30. Rodman, Toby C. et al. "Naturally Occurring Antibodies Reactive with Sperm Proteins: Apparent Deficiency in AIDS Sera." Science, v. 228, June 7, 1985, pp. 1211-1215.

It has been found that both males and females of all ages have naturally occurring antibodies to sperm proteins. These antibodies are significantly decreased in AIDS victims and may play a role in the development of AIDS.

31. Sattaur, Omar. "AIDS Victims Still Await Vaccine." New Scientist, v. 105, January 24, 1985, p. 20.

American and French scientists have found what is believed to be the entire gene sequence of the AIDS virus. An AIDS blood test is currently awaiting approval by the FDA.

32. Seale, John. "What We Know About AIDS." New Scientist, v. 107, August 1, 1985, pp. 29-30.

AIDS is a disease that destroys the immune system, leaving the body open to secondary infections that can kill the victim. It is caused by a lentivirus that destroys the cells it infects. AIDS is compared with similar blood-borne diseases in animals that have a high mortality rate.

33. Stevens, Cladd E. et al. "Human T-Cell Lymphotropic Virus Type III Infection in a Cohort of Homosexual Men in New York City." JAMA: Journal of the American Medical Association, v. 255, April 25, 1986, pp. 2167-2172.

Antibodies to the HTLV-III virus were examined in blood samples from 1978 to the present in 378 homosexual men. The percentages of men with antibodies has risen by 5% to 10% each year. Those men who had antibodies the longest showed significantly lower T-cell ratios.

34. "Toxoplasmosis and AIDS." American Family Physician, v. 31, February 1985, p. 345.

Toxoplasmosis, which is relatively rare, appears to have a high incidence in AIDS patients. Some methods to treat toxoplasmosis are given.

35. U.S. Centers for Disease Control. Reports on AIDS Published in the Morbidity and Mortality Weekly Report. Atlanta, GA: Centers for Disease Control, cumulated and issued quarterly. Superintendent of Documents Number HE20.7009/a:Ac7/.

A complete collection of articles dealing with AIDS published in the MMWR, including articles on epidemiology, secondary infection, transmission, and the spread of AIDS outside of the high risk groups.

36. Volberding, Paul A. "Kaposi's Sarcoma and the Acquired Immunodeficiency Syndrome." Medical Clinics of North America, v. 70, May 1986, pp. 665-676.

The clinical features of Kaposi's sarcoma as it relates to AIDS are described. Guidelines are given for the role of radiotherapy and chemotherapy in fighting Kaposi's sarcoma in AIDS patients.

37. Walgate, Robert. "New Human Retroviruses: One Causes AIDS..." Nature, v. 320, April 3, 1986, p. 385.

A second virus that can cause AIDS has been found that is at least 30% different in its gene sequence. This new virus has been named LAV-II by the French researchers who discovered it.

38. "World Health Organization Workshop: Conclusions and Recommendations on Acquired Immunodeficiency Syndrome." MMWR: Morbidity and Mortality Weekly Report, v. 34, May 17, 1985, pp. 275-276.

An international conference on AIDS sponsored by the World Health Organization and the U.S. Department of Health and Human Services resulted in a set of guidelines for the World Health Organization and its member countries to follow in dealing with AIDS. These guidelines are summarized.

39. Wormser, Gary P. "Multiple Opportunistic Infections and Neoplasms in the Acquired Immunodeficiency Syndrome." JAMA: Journal of the American Medical Association, v. 253, June 21, 1985, pp. 3441-3442.

AIDS is caused by a retrovirus, HTLV-III, and this infection leads to a destruction of the immune system. Other infections then occur, often multiple, and lead to death. Tissue cultures can be used to identify secondary infections, but the ideal management of AIDS must confront HTLV-III.

Epidemiology and Transmission

40. "AIDS Could Plague the World, Or Not." <u>New Scientist</u>, v. 105, February 14, 1985, p. 5.
   At present, it is impossible to predict how many cases of AIDS will be found in 1990. Because of the short history and rapid growth of the disease, the number may range anywhere from one to millions.

41. "AIDS: Counting the Bodies and the Antibodies." <u>New Scientist</u>, v. 108, October 3, 1985, p. 20.
   Over 12,000 people will contract AIDS during 1986. Most of the victims are homosexual men (73%), intravenous drug users (17%), blood transfusion recipients (22%), or female partners of men in high risk groups (1%). There are fewer cases outside of the United States, but these are also increasing rapidly.

42. "AIDS in Pregnancy, Donors, and Tears." <u>Science News</u>, v. 128, September 21, 1985, p. 187.
   New evidence indicates that AIDS may be exacerbated by pregnancy and that the virus may be transmitted through tears. The Centers for Disease Control have recommended that men with even a single homosexual experience since 1977 refrain from giving blood.

43. "AIDS Incidence Increases As Experts Continue Investigations." <u>American Family Physician</u>, v. 33, March 1986, pp. 328-329.
   As of January, 16,458 cases of AIDS have been reported. Over 50% of the victims have died and the number of cases is doubling every year. 65% of the victims are homosexual men, 17% are intravenous drug users, 8% are male homosexual drug users, 2% are recipients of blood transfusions, 1% are hemophiliacs, and 1% are heterosexual partners of AIDS victims. Six percent of the cases are unclassified.

44. "AIDS: Saliva Is Safe." <u>New Scientist</u>, v. 105, February 28, 1985, p. 7.
   There is no evidence that anyone has ever contracted AIDS by exposure to saliva. If the virus were spread in this manner many sporadic cases would appear in areas without other risk factors. This is not the case.

45. "AIDS Saliva Link Is Questioned." <u>New Scientist</u>, v. 105, February 14, 1985, p. 5.
   The AIDS virus may be present in saliva, but only in very minute amounts. It is extremely unlikely that AIDS is spread through kissing.

46. "AIDS Study Finds Virus Widespread." <u>New Scientist</u>, v. 106, April 25, 1985, p. 3.

One third of the homosexual men and 40% of hemophiliacs in London have been exposed to AIDS. Only 2.5% of intravenous drug users exhibited positive results.

47. "AIDS Toll Rises." <u>U.S. News and World Report</u>, v. 97, November 26, 1984, p. 80.

The number of AIDS victims doubled during 1984 and has now reached 6,857. Between 30 and 50 times as many people may be infected. It is spread through sexual contact and blood transfusions.

48. "AIDS Virus: Infection Up?" <u>Science News</u>, v. 128, November 23, 1985, p. 325.

A new estimate of AIDS infections puts the number of people with contact to the virus at two million.

49. Bennett, Jo Anne. "AIDS: Epidemiology Update." <u>American Journal of Nursing</u>, v. 85, September 1985, pp. 968-972.

Over 12,000 cases of AIDS have now been reported. It is transmitted through sexual contact, shared needles of drug users, or blood transfusions. In order to reduce the risk of contracting AIDS, it is important to engage only in safe sex without the exchange of bodily fluids with known partners. Drug users should use clean needles and pregnant women should discuss the risk of AIDS with a physician.

50. Castro, Kenneth G., Ann M. Hardy, and James W. Curran. "The Acquired Immunodeficiency Syndrome: Epidemiology and Risk Factors for Transmission." <u>Medical Clinics of North America</u>, v. 70, May 1986, pp. 635-650.

AIDS primarily affects young adults living in several metropolitan areas. Most patients are homosexual men, but heterosexual men and women who use intravenous drugs, who are hemophiliacs, or who are sexual partners of persons with AIDS are also at a high risk for AIDS.

51. Church, George J. "Not an Easy Disease to Come By." <u>Time</u>, v. 126, September 23, 1985, p. 27.

In contrast to the hysteria and fear related to AIDS, there are really only four ways to get the disease: by blood transfusion, shared hypodermic needles, childbirth, or sexual relations.

52. Curran, James W. et al. "The Epidemiology of AIDS: Current Status and Future Prospects." Science, v. 229, September 27, 1985, pp. 1352-1357.

The number of cases of AIDS is going to double every year, with over 12,000 cases reported in 1986. For single men in New York City and San Francisco between the ages of 25 and 44, AIDS is the leading cause of death. Many more people have been exposed to the virus than have contracted the disease. The use of blood screening should help to reduce the risk of infection via transfusion. Most infections occur through sexual contact, contaminated needles, or from mothers to infants.

53. Gauthier, Michael. "AIDS, Athletes, and Fears About Contact." Physician and Sportsmedicine, v. 14, January 1986, p. 41.

Some athletes and other participants in sports are worried about contracting AIDS through athletic contact. There is no evidence that such incidental contact causes AIDS.

54. Goedert, James J. et al. "Three-Year Incidence of AIDS in Five Cohorts of HTLV-III Infected Risk Group Members." Science, v. 231, February 28, 1986, pp. 992-995.

The three year incidence among HTLV-III seropositive high risk men revealed a rate of 34.2% for men from Manhattan and 14.9% for those from other localities. This may imply that the virus was introduced to New York before the rest of the country.

55. Hardy, Ann M. et al. "The Incidence Rate of Acquired Immunodeficiency Syndrome in Selected Populations." JAMA: Journal of the American Medical Association, v. 253, January 11, 1985, pp. 215-220.

Incidence rates of AIDS were determined for single men, intravenous drug users, Haitians, hemophiliacs, female sexual contacts of AIDS victims, and blood transfusion recipients. Single men in New York City and San Francisco, drug users in New York and New Jersey, hemophilia A patients, and recent Haitian immigrants had the highest rates of AIDS.

56. Kaplan, Jonathon E. "A Modern-Day Plague." Natural History, v. 95, February 1986, pp. 28-33.

AIDS is compared to other epidemics of the past. The AIDS infection rate is half that of polio in the 1950's, but among never-married men it is double the rate of chicken-pox. Because of the long lead time of the disease and the fact that we do not know how many people are infected, these rates are likely to rise during the next five years.

57. Marx, Jean L. "The Slow, Insidious Nature of the HTLV's." Science, v. 231, January 31, 1986, pp. 450-451.

Between 500,000 and one million people have been exposed to the AIDS virus and 5% to 10% of those will contract AIDS. Because of the long latency period, this estimate may be much too low. It is possible that some drugs may be developed to combat the virus.

58. Mayer, Kenneth H. "The Epidemiological Investigation of AIDS." Hastings Center Report, v. 15, August 1985, supplement pp. 12-15.

Studying epidemiology has been very useful in learning about AIDS. Following individuals who have changed their sexual habits may give clues as to the further spread of the disease. Studies may be hindered by the social intolerance of the primary groups. Epidemiological research may also raise some social questions, such as confidentiality of results and the quarantining of victims.

59. Meldrum, Julian. "How a Virus That Is Very Hard to Catch Crossed the World." New Statesman, v. 110, September 27, 1985, pp. 14-15.

AIDS probably originated with a virus that infects Green Monkeys in Africa. About fifteen years ago, it spread to Kinshasa and other urban African areas where it has been spread through people with many sexual partners. It was the transferred to the United States by gay men and blood transfusions. If no treatments are discovered, thousands of people of all ages and both sexes will die.

60. "No AIDS from Saliva." Newsweek, v. 106, December 30, 1985, p. 69.

There is very little evidence that AIDS can be transmitted by saliva. There are no known cases where it has been transmitted in this manner.

61. Norman, Colin. "AIDS Trends: Projections from Limited Data." Science, v. 230, November 29, 1985, pp. 1018-1021.

Almost everyone who gets AIDS belongs to one of the high risk groups. It is a very difficult disease to catch and requires direct insertion of the virus into the blood stream. There has been no change in the pattern of transmission, but the long latency period makes it difficult to determine.

62. Norman, Colin. "A Disease In Many Guises." Science, v. 230, November 29, 1985, p. 1019.

It is not clear if the millions of people exposed to the virus will actually contract AIDS. Many of these individuals are developing symptoms not generally associated with AIDS. Some long-term studies are needed.

63. "Number of AIDS Cases Likely to Escalate Rapidly." <u>Chemical and Engineering News</u>, v. 63, September 23, 1985, p. 5.

As many as one million Americans may have been exposed to the AIDS virus. Over 13,000 confirmed cases of AIDS have been reported so far and this number is expected to double every twelve months. The most common method of transmission is through sexual contact.

64. Peterman, Thomas A., D. Peter Drotman, and James W. Curran. "Epidemiology of the Acquired Immunodeficiency Syndrome (AIDS)." Epidemiological Reviews, v. 7, 1985, pp. 1-21.

AIDS is a deadly disease caused by the HTLV-III virus that attacks the immune system and leaves the body open to infection. AIDS is primarily limited to five high risk groups: homosexual men, intravenous drug users, Haitians, hemophiliacs, and female partners of infected men. In order to prevent the spread of the disease, it is important not to have sexual contact with infected individuals and blood should be screened for the AIDS virus.

65. "Reassuring the Families of AIDS Victims." <u>Newsweek</u>, v. 107, February 17, 1986, p. 78.

Evidence continues to mount to show that AIDS cannot be transmitted by casual contact. AIDS patients do not pose a risk to public health.

66. "Recommendations for Preventing Possible Transmission of Human T-Lymphotropic Virus Type III/Lymphadenopathy Associated Virus from Tears." <u>MMWR: Morbidity and Mortality Weekly Report</u>, v. 34, August 30, 1985, pp. 533-534.

The AIDS virus has recently been isolated from the tears of AIDS victims. Some guidelines are given for health and eye care personnel working with AIDS patients to avoid transmission of the virus.

67. "Results of a Gallup Poll on Acquired Immunodeficiency Syndrome: New York City, United States, 1985." <u>MMWR: Morbidity and Mortality Weekly Report</u>, v. 34, August 23, 1985, pp. 513-514.

The results of two Gallup polls on the groups most likely to have AIDS and its methods of transmission are reported. There were very few regional differences in the results, but individuals in low income groups seemed to be the least knowledgeable about the disease.

68. Servaas, Cory. "Help Prevent the Spread of AIDS." <u>Saturday Evening Post</u>, v. 258, January/February 1986, pp. 106-107.

In order to help prevent the spread of AIDS, we should not engage in promiscuous sexual activities or use illegal drugs. The blood supply is safer now, but to be entirely sure you should only accept blood from a known donor.

69. Silberner, Joanne. "AIDS: Casual Contact Exonerated." <u>Science News</u>, v. 128, October 5, 1985, p. 213.

AIDS is not transmitted by casual contact with a victim, but is being transmitted much more frequently through heterosexual contact.

70. Silberner, Joanne. "AIDS: Disease, Research Efforts Advance." <u>Science News</u>, v. 127, April 27, 1985, pp. 260-261.

The incidence of AIDS is increasing exponentially and it is spread primarily through intimate contact. Based on blood test results, one million people have been exposed to the virus. While researchers continue to look for a cure or vaccine, the disease continues to spread.

71. Silberner, Joanne. "New Directions in AIDS Transmission." <u>Science News</u>, v. 129, February 15, 1986, p. 101.

New studies on the transmission of AIDS reconfirm that casual contact does not cause AIDS. However, one case of a mother contracting AIDS from her child has been confirmed and a relation between clitoroidectomies and heterosexual transmission has been found in Africa.

72. Tanne, Janice H. "The Last Word on Avoiding AIDS." <u>New York</u>, v. 18, October 7, 1985, pp. 28-34.

Many people in New York are worried about contracting AIDS. Although many people have been exposed to the virus, the only way to catch AIDS is through sexual contact, intravenous drug use, or blood transfusions. There is no risk from casual contact with an AIDS victim.

73. "Threat of AIDS Widening to the General Public." <u>U.S. News and World Report</u>, v. 99, August 5, 1985, p. 66.

An interview with Dr. James Curran. AIDS is increasing daily and over 500,000 people have been exposed to the virus. The best way to reduce your chances of contracting AIDS is not to have sex with an infected person.

74. "Update: Acquired Immunodeficiency Syndrome in the San Francisco Cohort Study, 1978-1985." <u>MMWR: Morbidity and Mortality Weekly Report</u>, v. 34, September 27, 1985, pp. 573-575.

A group of 6,875 gay men who had enrolled in a sexually transmitted disease study between 1978 and 1980 were examined retrospectively for antibodies to the AIDS virus. Incidence of exposure rose from 4.5% in 1978 to 67.3% in 1984. The members of this group demonstrate the highest incidence rate in the United States.

75. "Update: Acquired Immunodeficiency Syndrome: United States." <u>MMWR: Morbidity and Mortality Weekly Report</u>, v. 34, May 10, 1985, pp. 245-248.

   Ten thousand confirmed cases of AIDS have now been reported, 9,887 adults and 113 children. The distribution of ages and proportion of victims in each high risk group have remained approximately the same.

76. "Update: Acquired Immunodeficiency Syndrome: United States." <u>MMWR: Morbidity and Mortality Weekly Report</u>, v. 35, January 17, 1986, pp. 17-21.

   Over 16,000 cases of AIDS have been reported as of January 13, 1986. Statistics on adult and child cases are provided. The number of new cases is expected to rise more slowly in 1986 than it did in 1985.

77. Wallis, Claudia. "Lessening Fears." <u>Time</u>, v. 127, February 17, 1986, p. 90.

   New research supports the findings that there is no risk of contracting AIDS through casual contact. It cannot be transmitted in families, schools, offices, restaurants, or churches.

78. "Workers and AIDS: Uncle Sam Speaks." <u>U.S. News and World Report</u>, v. 99, November 25, 1985, p. 14.

   The Public Health Service has issued an official statement saying that AIDS is not transmitted by casual contact. Some specific safety guidelines for health-care workers, barbers and hairdressers, and food service workers are included.

AIDS, the Blood Supply, and the AIDS Blood Test

79. "AIDS Antibody Screening Test." <u>Analytical Chemistry</u>, v. 57, June 1985, pp. 773A-777A.

The enzyme linked immunosorbent assay (ELISA) test for AIDS antibodies has been developed. This test is easy and inexpensive to run but it has a tendency to produce false positive results. It also does not indicate the presence of the virus, only past exposure. However, it should be useful in screening blood donors.

80. "AIDS in Hemophiliacs." <u>American Family Physician</u>, v. 32, July 1985, p. 222.

The number of cases of AIDS associated with hemophilia appears to be stabilizing or even declining. Statistics related to AIDS in hemophiliacs are provided.

81. "AIDS Update." <u>Scientific American</u>, v. 252, April 1985, p. 70.

The AIDS virus is a retrovirus called either HTLV-III or LAV. The full nucleotide sequence has just been discovered. A new blood test should keep the virus out of the blood supply, but does not positively identify those carrying the AIDS virus.

82. "Amid the Debate Over AIDS Tests, Some Progress." <u>Discover</u>, v. 6, March 1985, p. 12.

An AIDS blood test is just over the horizon, but it is not entirely accurate. Gay rights groups are worried that the test will be used to discriminate against homosexual men.

83. "Bad Blood?" <u>Scientific American</u>, v. 252, December 1985, pp. 78-79.

The AIDS blood tests may not make the blood supply safe. One study indicates that at least 5% of blood samples carrying the AIDS virus escape detection by the ELISA test.

84. Barber, John et al. "The Indiscriminate Killer." <u>Macleans</u>, v. 98, August 12, 1985, p. 38.

Many people are afraid of catching AIDS through blood transfusions. The development of a new blood test to screen all donated blood samples should eliminate this method of spreading AIDS.

85. Beardsley, Tim. "U.S. Blood-Bank Test Established." <u>Nature</u>, v. 316, August 8, 1985, p. 474.

The first second-generation AIDS blood test has just been developed. This test detects viral antigens in blood rather than their antibodies and avoids many of the false positive results of the ELISA test.

86. Budiansky, Stephen. "AIDS Tests Alarm Blood Banks." <u>Nature</u>, v. 313, January 10, 1985, p. 87.

The American Association of Blood Banks has recommended that the new blood tests be run on every unit of blood collected. Some blood bank officials are worried about the high false-positive rate for test results.

87. Budiansky, Stephen. "Blood Test Trials Inconclusive." <u>Nature</u>, v. 316, July 11, 1985, p. 96.

The new ELISA blood test still raises some concern. It has a tendency to produce false positive results. This test will now be compared to results from other testing methods.

88. Carlson, James R. et al. "AIDS Serology Testing in Low- and High-Risk Groups." <u>JAMA: Journal of the American Medical Association</u>, v. 253, June 21, 1985, pp. 3405-3408.

The ELISA, Western Blot, and immunofluorescence tests were all used on a group of over 1,000 blood samples. The ELISA test had a high false positive rate and should be backed by a confirmation test by one of the other two methods.

89. Chang, N. T. et al. "An HTLV-III Peptide Produced By Recombinant DNA Is Immunoreactive with Sera from Patients with AIDS." <u>Nature</u>, v. 315, May 9, 1985, pp. 151-154.

The sera of AIDS victims contains antibodies to the HTLV-III virus. A genetically engineered peptide encoded with a gene segment from HTLV-III may be useful in detecting the AIDS virus in blood samples.

90. "Changing Patterns of Acquired Immunodeficiency Syndrome in Hemophilia Patients: United States." <u>MMWR: Morbidity and Mortality Weekly Reports</u>, v. 34, May 3, 1985, pp. 241-243.

The number of hemophilia-associated AIDS cases appears to be stabilizing or even declining. The characteristics of new cases also appears to be changing, with almost 50% of the new cases involving individuals with disorders other than hemophilia A.

91. Clark, Matt and Pamela Abramson. "AIDS: The Blood-Bank Scare." <u>Newsweek</u>, v. 105, January 28, 1985, p. 62.

Many people are refusing to receive blood from a blood bank out of fear of contracting AIDS. Although the risks are extremely minimal, some patients will accept blood only from known donors.

92. Clarke, Maxine. "Two British Blood Tests Launched." Nature, v. 316, August 8, 1985, p. 474.

Five different AIDS blood tests have been examined and the British government has approved two for use in that country. Both of these are of the ELISA type.

93. Clarke, Maxine. "U.S. Company Rejects U.K. Decision." Nature, v. 316, August 29, 1985, p. 759.

Abbott Laboratories, the manufacturer of an AIDS blood test, is protesting the decision of British health officials to use a competing company's test. The lab feels that the British survey results are preliminary and misleading.

94. Connor, Steve. "Blood Treatment May Not Kill AIDS Virus." New Scientist, v. 109, February 20, 1986, pp. 13-14.

AIDS will become the biggest health problem in Britain in this century. Recent evidence indicates that heat treatment used on blood samples may not be entirely successful in killing the AIDS virus. Different blood companies use different techniques, none of which has been shown to be 100% effective.

95. Curran, William J. "AIDS Research and the Window of Opportunity." New England Journal of Medicine, v. 312, April 4, 1985, pp. 903-904.

A forthcoming blood test for AIDS antibodies raises a number of legal questions. Any donors who test positive should be notified of that result. To avoid false positives, a second test should be run. Anyone receiving AIDS-contaminated blood should also be notified.

96. Eckert, Rose D. "AIDS and the Blood Supply." Consumer Research Magazine, v. 68, October 1985, pp. 20-25.

AIDS is a deadly disease that has been associated with blood transfusions. This virus is a threat to the national blood supply. Many individuals are only accepting blood from known donors until an effective screening method is discovered.

97. Fierman, Jacalyn. "Helping Battle AIDS." Fortune, v. 111, April 15, 1985, pp. 57-58.

Five companies are competing to develop a blood test for the AIDS virus. The test will determine if antibodies to the virus are present, but not the virus itself.

98. Finlayson, Ann. "Testing Donors for AIDS." Macleans, v. 98, May 27, 1985, p. 49.

Two people who contracted AIDS through blood transfusions in Vancouver have caused the Canadian Red Cross to begin testing blood donors for the AIDS virus. Even though the chances of getting AIDS through blood transfusions are minimal, this test should help to keep the blood supply free of the virus.

99. Goldsmith, Marsha F. "HTLV-III Testing of Donor Blood Imminent: Complex Issues Remain." JAMA: Journal of the American Medical Association, v. 253, January 11, 1985, pp. 173-181.

Testing of blood for antibodies to the AIDS virus will soon begin. While this test will protect the nation's blood supply, it does not mean that any individual has the virus. The civil rights of those groups most at risk must be protected.

100. "High Exposure." Time, v. 127, March 24, 1986, p. 35.

Government officials have suggested that millions of individuals in the high risk groups be tested for antibodies to the AIDS virus. Some people are worried that such a mass screening would be used to discriminate against homosexuals.

101. "How Blood Traders Could Have Launched AIDS." New Scientist, v. 105, March 28, 1985, p. 7.

A new theory on the origin of AIDS is that the virus was spread to the United States by illicit blood dealers. These blood dealers buy cheap plasma in Africa and the Caribbean and resell it at inflated prices in the U.S. This theory does not correlate with the fact that AIDS was identified in hemophiliacs only after it was found in homosexuals.

102. "Isolation of Human T-Lymphotropic Virus Type III/Lymphadenopathy Associated Virus from Serum Proteins Given to Cancer Patients: Bahamas." MMWR: Morbidity and Mortality Weekly Reports, v. 34, August 9, 1985, pp. 489-491.

A controversial cancer treatment that is not approved in the United States involves the reinjection of the patient's own blood serum. An evaluation of this method as practiced in the Bahamas indicates that the serum has helped to spread AIDS.

103. Jason, Janine et al. "Human T-Lymphotropic Retrovirus Type III/Lymphadenopathy-Associated Virus Antibody." JAMA: Journal of the American Medical Association, v. 253, June 21, 1985, pp. 3409-3415.

Approximately 400 persons routinely receiving blood transfusions were studied for antibodies to the AIDS virus. It appears that both blood factors VIII and IX may transmit the AIDS virus.

104. Johnstone, Bob. "New AIDS Test Comes to Light in Japan." New Scientist, v. 106, April 18, 1985, p. 8.

A new test for AIDS developed in Japan is cheaper and more reliable than the Western Blot method. It uses a fluorescence microscope to spot antibodies to the AIDS virus. However, up to 10% of the samples can falsely be diagnosed as positive and must be retested.

105. Landesman, Sheldon H., Harold M. Ginzburg, and Stanley W. Weiss. "The AIDS Epidemic." New England Journal of Medicine, v. 312, February 21, 1985, pp. 521-525.

Several important developments have been made in the understanding of AIDS. The ELISA blood test can detect antibodies to the HTLV-III virus. This test and other studies indicate that large numbers of people will become infected and thousands will die. The disease will also have tremendous economic, social, and ethical considerations.

106. Levine, Carol and Ronald Bayer. "Screening Blood: Public Health and Medical Uncertainty." Hastings Center Report, v. 15, August 1985, supplement pp. 8-11.

Fears of a contaminated blood supply led to the development of the ELISA test for exposure to HTLV-III. This test measures the presence of antibodies to the virus but does not confirm the presence of AIDS. It has problems in that it produces false positive results. Two ethical questions related to the test are its use in mass screening of selected populations and the reporting of results to the individuals and/or outside parties.

107. Marwick, Charles. "Use of AIDS Antibody Test May Provide More Answers." JAMA: Journal of the American Medical Association, v. 253, March 22, 1985, pp. 1694-1699.

The ELISA blood test will enable researchers to conduct further epidemiological studies on AIDS. This test detects antibodies to the AIDS virus to a 95% specificity.

108. McDonald, Marc. "A Startling AIDS-Related Discovery." Macleans, v. 98, July 15, 1985, pp. 42-43.

A Canadian researcher has applied for a patent on a method of purifying hemoglobin which greatly reduces the risk of transmitting AIDS. This same procedure could also lead to the freeze-drying of blood supplies.

109. Miller, Roger W. "The Reasons Behind Blood Donor Screening." FDA Consumer, v. 19, November 1985, pp. 31-34.

Contamination of blood by the AIDS virus is only the latest in a series of efforts to prevent the spread of disease through blood transfusions. Questions about the transmission of AIDS and other symptoms are answered.

110. "Ministers Delayed Launch of AIDS Test." New Scientist, v. 107, August 8, 1985, p. 16.

The British government delayed in approving an AIDS screening test until one was developed in Britain. While American blood supplies have kept AIDS-free, British supplies could be contaminated because of the lack of testing.

111. Norman, Colin. "FDA Approves Pasteur's AIDS Test Kit." Science, v. 231, March 7, 1986, p. 1063.

The FDA has approved a French blood test for AIDS antibodies. This may add fuel to the French claim to patent rights to the virus.

112. Peterman, Thomas A. "Transfusion-Associated Acquired Immunodeficiency Syndrome in the United States." JAMA: Journal of the American Medical Association, v. 254, November 22, 1985, pp. 2913-2917.

By August 15, 1985, 194 cases of AIDS resulting from blood transfusions had been reported. Infants accounted for 10% of the cases, suggesting a higher susceptibility. The risk of contracting AIDS from blood transfusions is low and will be lowered even further by blood screening.

113. Peterson, Faye. "Screening Blood Donations for AIDS." FDA Consumer, v. 19, May 1985, pp. 5-11.

Some questions about AIDS are answered, including how it is transmitted, what the AIDS blood test results mean, and how the blood supply is protected against AIDS.

114. "Provisional Public Health Service Inter-Agency Recommendations for Screening Donated Blood and Plasma for Antibody to the Virus Causing Acquired Immunodeficiency Syndrome." MMWR: Morbidity and Mortality Weekly Report, v. 34, January 11, 1985, pp. 1-5.

The ELISA blood test allows for the effective screening of blood donations for antibodies to the AIDS virus. Recommendations are given for both blood banks and blood donors regarding the proper ethical and safety procedures in the screening of blood donations.

115. "Results of Human T-Lymphotropic Virus Type III Test Kits Reported from Blood Collection Centers: United States, April 22-May 19, 1985." MMWR: Morbidity and Mortality Weekly Reports, v. 34, June 28, 1985, pp. 375-376.

The ELISA blood test was examined for its effectiveness in examining 593,831 units of blood. It showed an initial result of 0.89% reactive, of which 0.25% were found to be reactive in subsequent tests.

116. Rock, Andrea. "Inside the Billion-Dollar Business of Blood." Money, v. 15, March 1986, pp. 152-172.

Blood banks were slow to recognize that AIDS could be transmitted by transfusions and were slow to come up with a test to examine blood for the AIDS virus. A detailed account of how the blood industry reacted to the AIDS crisis is presented.

117. Sattaur, Omar. "AIDS Tests Could Trigger World Blood Shortage." New Scientist, v. 106, May 16, 1985, p. 6.
    The new AIDS blood tests will have a significant effect on the world's blood supply. False positive results will cause good blood to be wasted and false-negative results will contaminate otherwise usable blood supplies. The social consequences of blood testing have yet to be determined.

118. Sattaur, Omar. "New British Test for AIDS Is Quicker and Cheaper." New Scientist, v. 108, October 3, 1985, pp. 20-21.
    A new British AIDS blood test will help to solve the problem of false-positive results. This test will now become the standard British blood test.

119. Sattaur, Omar. "Sharper Tests for AIDS." New Scientist, v. 106, May 2, 1985, p. 23.
    A new testing method called ELISA (enzyme-linked immunosorbent assay) is able to test for AIDS antibodies without creating false positives or negatives. By using biotechnology to create sufficient amounts of AIDS proteins, false results can be eliminated.

120. Silberner, Joanne. "AIDS Blood Test: Qualified Success." Science News, v. 128, August 10, 1985, p. 84.
    The new AIDS blood test is very good at identifying AIDS-infected blood, but it also has a tendency to produce false positive results, especially in the blood of women. Several companies are working on a more accurate second-generation test.

121. Silberner, Joanne. "The Great AIDS Race: Testing the Test." Science News, v. 127, January 19, 1985, p. 36.
    Five companies have submitted AIDS blood tests for approval to the FDA. The decision on which tests to use is due at any time. The availability of such a test will help to prevent the transmission of AIDS through the nation's blood supply.

122. Spencer, Norman. "Medical Anthropology and the AIDS Epidemic: A Case Study in San Francisco." Urban Anthropology, v. 12, Summer 1983, pp. 141-159.
    The decision to take the test for antibodies to the AIDS virus is very complex. How the test results are received and acted upon is also a complex cultural and psychosocial process. These issues are examined from an anthropological viewpoint.

123. Swinbanks, David. "Japan Screens Donated Blood." Nature, v. 319, February 20, 1986, p. 610.
    Japan's Health and Welfare Ministry has begun to test blood donations for the AIDS virus. Although the government does not feel that it is worth the expense, they will test blood anyway to alleviate public fears.

124. Swinbanks, David. "Undesirable Import to Japan." <u>Nature</u>, v. 315, May 2, 1985, p. 8.

Two Japanese hemophiliacs have died of AIDS that they probably contracted through contaminated blood imported from the United States. Despite the risk of AIDS, blood imports will continue and no screening program will be implemented.

125. Teitelman, Robert. "Leveraging AIDS." <u>Forbes</u>, v. 135, April 8, 1985, p. 115.

Biotechnology companies are in a race to develop a blood test for AIDS. At stake is a $170 million worldwide market.

126. "U.S. Prepares for AIDS Blood Test." <u>New Scientist</u>, v. 105, January 17, 1985, p. 3.

The U.S. government has asked members of the four high risk groups to refrain from donating blood. A new blood test for antibodies to the AIDS virus should be available later in the year.

127. "Update: Public Health Service Workshop on Human T-Lymphotropic Virus Type III Antibody Testing: United States." <u>MMWR: Morbidity and Mortality Weekly Reports</u>, v. 34, August 9, 1985, pp. 477-478.

Of 1.1 million units of blood tested with the ELISA blood test, 0.25% of the results have repeatedly been positive. Those blood samples that are strongly positive with the ELISA test are usually also positive with other test methods, but those that are weekly positive are not good indicators of the presence of the virus.

128. "Update: Revised Public Health Service Definition of Persons Who Should Refrain from Donating Blood and Plasma: United States." <u>MMWR: Morbidity and Mortality Weekly Reports</u>, v. 34, September 6, 1985, pp. 547-548.

The Food and Drug Administration has revised the wording of its donor-referral recommendations to add men who have had even a single homosexual contact since 1977 to its list of those who should not donate blood.

129. "Virologists Discount Fear of AIDS in Hepatitis B Vaccine." <u>New Scientist</u>, v. 108, November 7, 1985, p. 21.

There appears to be absolutely no risk that the Hepatitis B vaccine can transmit AIDS. This concern arose because homosexual men often carry Hepatitis B and the vaccine is made from their blood sera.

130. Walgate, Robert. "France to Screen Blood Donors." <u>Nature</u>, v. 315, June 27, 1985, p. 705.

France will soon require testing of all blood donors for the AIDS virus. It is not yet clear if donors will be informed, but the cost will be $30 million per year.

131. Weiss, Stanley H. et al. "Screening Test for HTLV-III (AIDS Agent) Antibodies: Specificity, Sensitivity, and Applications." <u>JAMA: Journal of the American Medical Association</u>, v. 253, January 11, 1985, pp. 221-225.

In a test of the enzyme-linked immunosorbent assay (ELISA), 98% of AIDS patients scored positive or borderline and 99% of control subjects scored negative. This will be a useful test for screening blood donors and populations at risk for AIDS.

132. Yanchinski, Stephanie. "AIDS Diagnosis Uncertain." <u>New Scientist</u>, v. 105, February 7, 1985, p. 24.

A blood test for AIDS is now available. Because the test only indicates the presence of antibodies to the virus, its usefulness is questionable. The primary use will be to test blood supplies in blood banks.

133. Yanchinski, Stephanie. "British Anti-AIDS Invention Sold Abroad." <u>New Scientist</u>, v. 107, August 8, 1985, p. 17.

Speywood Laboratories has developed a genetically engineered factor VIII, which is a blood clotting protein used in the treatment of hemophiliacs. The use of this genetically engineered product will reduce the risk of AIDS contamination in donated blood.

AIDS and Intravenous Drug Users

134. Caputo, Larry. "Dual Diagnosis: AIDS and Addiction." Social Work, v. 30, July/August 1985, pp. 360-364.

The second largest group commonly identified with AIDS are intravenous drug users. AIDS has many specific social and psychological effects on this group. The roles of social workers in dealing with this situation are explained.

135. Ginzburg, Harold M. "Intravenous Drug Users and the Acquired Immune Deficiency Syndrome." Public Health Reports, v. 99, March/April 1984, pp. 206-212.

Not only is the heroin user at risk for AIDS, but also the occasional recreational drug user who shares a needle to self-administer cocaine or amphetamines. Several million drug users may be at risk. Although drug treatment staffs are also concerned about AIDS, no cases of the transmission of AIDS to health care workers have been documented.

136. Koplan, Jeffrey P., Ann M. Hardy, and James R. Allen. "Epidemiology of the Acquired Immunodeficiency Syndrome in Intravenous Drug Abusers." Advances in Alcohol and Substance Abuse, v. 5, Fall/Winter 1985-1986, pp. 13-22.

Of the 3,694 reported cases of AIDS, 640 involved heterosexual intravenous drug users and 326 were homosexual intravenous drug users. The epidemiology of AIDS among drug users is described.

137. Pincus, Harold A. "AIDS, Drug Abuse, and Mental Health." Public Health Reports, v. 99, March/April 1984, pp. 106-108.

Intravenous drug users are a major risk group for AIDS. The interrelationship of behavioral and biological variables may be studied in this group. Research is needed to determine the behavioral factors involved in the spread of the disease and what behavior changes can be made to stop it.

138. Shine, Daniel. "Diagnosis and Management of Acquired Immune Deficiency Syndrome in Intravenous Drug Abusers." Advances in Alcohol and Substance Abuse, v. 5, Fall/Winter 1985-1986, pp. 25-34.

In drug users, AIDS almost always presents an opportunistic infection, usually Pneumocystis carinii. Recent research on AIDS in drug abusers is presented along with suggestions for the management of intravenous drug users with severe immune dysfunction.

AIDS Outside of the High Risk Groups

139. "AIDS (con't.)" <u>Science News</u>, v. 127, May 25, 1985, p. 328.

AIDS may be transmitted from mother to child through breast milk, the AIDS virus may have a much longer lead time, and the virus may be much more prevalent than previously thought.

140. "AIDS: How Real Is the Risk for Women?" <u>Glamour</u>, v. 83, November 1985, pp. 308-310.

It is possible to get AIDS through sexual intercourse or anal sex, but not through kissing. If a partner is bisexual or has had past homosexual contacts, the risk will be higher.

141. "AIDS: Probing the Heterosexual Link." <u>New Scientist</u>, v. 107, September 19, 1985, p. 15.

Of 76 men tested with AIDS antibodies, three of their female partners also exhibited antibodies. Although this indicates that the disease can be transmitted through heterosexual contact, it is not transmitted as easily as other sexually transmitted diseases.

142. "Apparent Transmission of Human T-Lymphotropic Virus Type III/Lymphadenopathy Associated Virus from a Child to a Mother Providing Health Care." <u>MMWR: Morbidity and Mortality Weekly Report</u>, v. 35, February 7, 1986, pp. 76-79.

A child who had contracted AIDS through blood transfusions may be responsible for his mother also contracting the disease. Because of her contact with the child's blood and bodily fluids, she may have accidentally injected the virus into her bloodstream.

143. Breu, Giovanna. "In New Jersey A Pediatrician Tends the Littlest Victims." <u>People</u>, v. 23, June 17, 1985, pp. 46-48.

Over 125 children under age thirteen have contracted AIDS. Dr. James Oleske is a pediatrician who specializes in AIDS victims.

144. Conant, Jennet and Linda R. Prout. "AIDS: A Link with Poverty?" <u>Newsweek</u>, v. 105, June 24, 1985, p. 37.

Belle Glade, Florida has the highest incidence of AIDS in the country and many of the cases do not fall into the high risk categories. This high rate may be somehow linked to the extreme poverty and squalid conditions of the residents.

145. Echenberg, Dean F. "A New Strategy to Prevent the Spread of AIDS Among Heterosexuals." <u>JAMA: Journal of the American Medical Association</u>, v. 154, October 18, 1985, pp. 2129-2130.

An educational campaign is being used to alert the heterosexual population about AIDS. The practice of safer sex is the only way to stop the spread of the disease.

146. Goldsmith, Marsha. "More Heterosexual Spread of HTLV-III Virus Seen." <u>JAMA: Journal of the American Medical Association</u>, v. 253, June 21, 1985, pp. 3377-3379.

There is mounting evidence that AIDS may be spread by heterosexual contact. Some cases of males outside the high risk groups who contracted AIDS from females with AIDS are documented.

147. Groocock, Veronica. "Scare Hits Women, Not Gay Men Alone." <u>New Statesman</u>, v. 110, August 30, 1985, pp. 12-13.

Some women are beginning to fear the risk of contracting AIDS. Many women who were married to bisexual men have gotten divorced or separated or have simply stopped having sex with their husbands.

148. "Haitians and AIDS." <u>American Family Physician</u>, v. 31, June 1985, p. 241.

Haitian immigrants have been removed from the list of high risk groups for AIDS. Only 3% of all cases involve Haitians.

149. "Heterosexual Transmission of Human T-Lymphotropic Virus Type III/Lymphadenopathy Associated Virus." <u>MMWR: Morbidity and Mortality Weekly Report</u>, v. 34, September 20, 1985, pp. 561-563.

Over one hundred sexual partners of AIDS victims who do not belong to any other high risk groups have contracted AIDS. This indicates a possible heterosexual link in the transmission of the virus.

150. "Heterosexuals Too Are at Risk." <u>People</u>, v. 23, June 17, 1985, p. 45.

Some questions and answers about AIDS. The virus can be spread to heterosexuals through sexual contact, but not through casual contact. There are currently no successful treatments or vaccines.

151. Jayaraman, K. S. "Pool of Infected Women?" <u>Nature</u>, v. 321, May 8, 1986, p. 103.

The Indian government is expanding its AIDS surveillance after discovering six cases of AIDS in female prostitutes. It is feared that these women have spread the disease to their male contacts.

152. Martin, Thad. "AIDS: Is It a Major Threat to Blacks?" <u>Ebony</u>, v. 40, October 1985, pp. 91-96.

AIDS occurs with a greater frequency in blacks than among other ethnic groups. Many blacks see AIDS as a "gay white disease" and are afraid to face the stigma associated with it. One reason AIDS may be more prevalent among blacks is that it is an urban disease and blacks are disproportionately urban.

153. McCoy, Kathy. "What You Should Know About AIDS." <u>Seventeen</u>, v. 44, November 1985, pp. 24-32.

AIDS is a disease that suppresses the immune system and is found primarily in homosexual men and drug users. Women are beginning to get AIDS and a blood test now exists to test for antibodies to the AIDS virus. It is transmitted either through sexual contact or blood transfusions.

154. Norwood, Christopher. "AIDS Is Not for Men Only." <u>Mademoiselle</u>, v. 91, September 1985, pp. 198-199+.

AIDS has hit 731 American women by mid-1985. It is spread by sexual contact, blood transfusion, or shared needles. In Africa, the ratio of women to men with AIDS is one to one. Safer sexual practices and care in choosing a partner will help prevent the spread of AIDS.

155. Pahwa, Savita et al. "Spectrum of Human T-Cell Lymphotropic Virus Type III Infection in Children." <u>JAMA: Journal of the American Medical Association</u>, v. 255, May 2, 1986, pp. 2299-2305.

In 36 children with HTLV infection, a wide clinical spectrum was seen, from fourteen children with AIDS to seven asymptomatic children. All twenty mothers studied showed antibodies to HTLV-III, but only nine were symptomatic. Apparently healthy women may transmit the AIDS virus to their children.

156. "Perinatal AIDS." <u>American Family Physician</u>, v. 33, February 1986, pp. 364-369.

The Centers for Disease Control have issued guidelines to pregnant women in high risk groups in order to prevent the spread of AIDS to newborns. The ELISA blood test is recommended for those women.

157. "Recommendations for Assisting in the Prevention of Perinatal Transmission of Human T-Lymphotropic Virus Type III/Lymphadenopathy Associated Virus and Acquired Immunodeficiency Syndrome." <u>MMWR: Morbidity and Mortality Weekly Report</u>, v. 34, December 6, 1985, pp. 721-732.

Three-fourths of all AIDS cases in children under thirteen years of age have mothers with AIDS as the only risk factor. Specific guidelines are included for educating and counseling women with AIDS who are pregnant or desire to have a child.

158. Redfield, Robert R. et al. "Heterosexually Acquired HTLV-III/LAV Disease (AIDS-Related Complex and AIDS)." <u>JAMA: Journal of the American Medical Association</u>, v. 254, October 18, 1985, pp. 2094-2096.

Of patients examined at the Walter Reed Army Medical Center, 37% contracted the AIDS virus from a partner of the opposite sex. This provides further evidence for the bidirectional heterosexual transmission of the disease.

159. Sattaur, Omar. "New Fears That Children May Catch AIDS." New Scientist, v. 106, April 18, 1985, p. 4.

Many more children may have AIDS than previously reported. Of children with AIDS, 74% are black or Hispanic and only 58% are male. Children may contract AIDS through the placenta, through the amniotic sac, or through direct contact with the vaginal walls.

160. Scott, Gwendolyn B. et al. "Mothers of Infants with the Acquired Immunodeficiency Syndrome: Evidence for Both Symptomatic and Asymptomatic Carriers." JAMA: Journal of the American Medical Association, v. 253, January 18, 1985, pp. 363-366.

Sixteen mothers of infants with AIDS were studied. Evidence indicates that mothers are the likely source of non-transfusion associated AIDS or AIDS-related-complex in infants.

161. Silberner, Joanne. "Female-to-Male AIDS Link Found." Science News, v. 129, March 15, 1986, pp. 164-165.

The AIDS virus has been found in the vaginal and cervical secretions of women who have antibodies to the virus. This may allow for female to male transmission of the disease.

162. Switzer, Ellen. "AIDS: What Women Can Do." Vogue, v. 176, January 1986, pp. 222-223+.

AIDS has spread quickly throughout the United States and is beginning to infect more women. It is spread only by blood or sex and care is cautioned in choosing sexual partners. The recent blood test determines exposure to the virus, not infection with the disease. AIDS is highly infectious, but not very contagious.

163. "To Stop AIDS." Health, v. 17, December 1985, p. 64.

AIDS has recently been spread to women by infected men. The only way to stop the spread of the disease is to carefully select sexual partners and practice defensive living.

164. Zimmerman, David R. "AIDS: What Women Must Know Now!" Good Housekeeping, v. 201, November 1985, pp. 245-246.

AIDS is spread primarily through sexual contact, drug abuse, or blood transfusions. The number of cases in women is rising and it is recommended that women engage in fewer casual sexual contacts. A blood test is now available for exposure to the virus, but it cannot indicate if any one individual will contract the disease.

The Search for an AIDS Cure

165. Anderson, Ian. "Black Market Forces Legalization of AIDS Drug." New Scientist, v. 106, May 16, 1985, p. 6.

Desperate AIDS victims are travelling to Mexico to buy two experimental drugs: isoprinosine and ribavirin. Because of this demand the FDA has eased restrictions on isoprinosine. There is still no evidence that it actually helps AIDS patients and clinical trials will not be completed until 1986.

166. Beardsley, Tim. "Aids: U.S. Law Delays Drug Testing." Nature, v. 317, October 17, 1985, p. 568.

Plans to speed up the clinical trials of some experimental AIDS drugs have been thwarted by a legal technicality. The National Institute for Allergy and Infectious Diseases had wanted to issue contracts to nine research centers to test the treatments, but this action is illegal under the Competition Act.

167. Beardsley, Tim. "Synthetic Vaccine Only a Distant Prospect." Nature, v. 314, April 25, 1985, p. 659.

The AIDS virus may recently have been transmitted to humans from monkeys. The best hope for stopping the disease is a vaccine against the virus, but this is still many years away. Antibodies to the virus have been found in a high percentage of hemophiliacs and promiscuous male homosexuals. All U.S. blood banks are now screening for AIDS.

168. Beauchamp, Marc. "AIDS to the Rescue?" Forbes, v. 136, November 18, 1985, pp. 72-74.

Isoprinosine may be effective against the AIDS virus, but it has not been approved for use by the FDA. The drug may help to strengthen the immune system, but the government claims to see no evidence for this.

169. Blaun, Randi. "Insurance Against AIDS?" New York, v. 18, June 3, 1985, pp. 62-65.

The drug isoprinosine has the ability to stimulate a weakened immune system. Although it does not cure a person of AIDS, it can keep the patient from getting worse. The FDA has not yet approved the drug for general usage.

170. Clark, Matt. "AIDS: A Breakthrough?" Newsweek, v. 106, November 11, 1985, p. 88.

The announcement by French scientists that a new drug is available to fight AIDS, cyclosporine, may be premature. Many scientists believe that not enough testing had been done before it was given to AIDS patients.

171. Clark, Matt. "AIDS Exiles in Paris." Newsweek, v. 106, August 5, 1985, p. 71.
 Some desperate AIDS patients, including Rock Hudson, have moved to Paris to try an experimental drug that is unavailable in the United States. The drug, HPA-23, appears to inhibit the viral activity but does not stop the disease once it affects the immune system. Some other experimental drugs are also discussed.

172. Clark, Matt. "AIDS Therapy: A Step Closer?" Newsweek, v. 107, February 24, 1986, p. 60.
 The crucial step in the reproduction of the AIDS virus is the translation of RNA into protein. It may be possible to stop the spread of AIDS by finding a drug that inhibits this process.

173. Davis, Jeff. "Desperate American AIDS Victims Journey to Paris, Hoping That a New Drug Can Stave Off Death." People, v. 24, August 12, 1985, pp. 42-43.
 Many AIDS victims, including Rock Hudson, are traveling to Paris to try the experimental drug HPA-23. This drug, which is a combination of tungsten and antimony, is not available in the United States.

174. Davis, L. "AIDS Vaccine Research: Promising Protein." Science News, v. 129, March 8, 1986, p. 151.
 A viral antigen from the outer coat or envelope of the AIDS virus may be useful in developing an AIDS vaccine. The earliest that such a vaccine would be available is 1988.

175. "Early Results Show Drug Helps Patients to Fight AIDS." New Scientist, v. 109, March 20, 1986, p. 23.
 A short trial of the drug azidothymidine has shown encouraging results for AIDS patients. After six weeks, fifteen of the nineteen subjects showed an increase in T-cells and a gain in body weight.

176. "Etoposide in AIDS Therapy." American Family Physician, v. 31, March 1985, p. 276.
 The drug etoposide has shown some success in treating Kaposi's sarcoma related to AIDS. While it does not prevent infection, it can keep the cancer in remission.

177. Francis, Donald P. and John C. Petricciani. "The Prospects for and Pathways Toward a Vaccine for AIDS." New England Journal of Medicine, v. 313, December 19, 1985, pp. 1586-1590.
 AIDS is caused by the HTLV-III/LAV virus. Some vaccines exist for other naturally occurring retroviruses, so there is hope that one can be developed for AIDS. Using a killed virus vaccine, testing can be conducted on chimpanzees and then humans. When developed, it should be administered to everyone in the high risk groups.

178. Goldsmith, Marsha F. "Not There Yet, But 'On Our Way' in AIDS Research." JAMA: Journal of the American Medical Association, v. 253, June 21, 1985, pp. 369-371+.

Despite the vast amount of information found out about AIDS, we still do not have a treatment or a cure. The only real means of eliminating the disease is to attack the HTLV-III virus. Several drugs have been attempted, but none has been entirely successful.

179. Haller, Scot. "An Angry New York Doctor Turns South-of-the-Border Smuggler to Treat Patients in Danger of AIDS." People, v. 24, October 14, 1985, pp. 139-142.

Dr. Barry Gingell made a trip to Mexico to purchase two experimental drugs used to treat AIDS patients, isoprinosine and ribavirin. Neither of the drugs are available in the United States. While there is no evidence that they help with AIDS, they do work on the AIDS-related-complex.

180. Heneson, Nancy. "When Will We Have an AIDS Vaccine?" New Scientist, v. 109, March 27, 1986, p. 20.

A vaccine against AIDS should be in the testing stage by 1988. Four steps need to be taken before then. We need to find out which parts of the virus stimulate immune response, the virus needs to be tested in animals, these tests must be rerun with Rhesus monkeys, and the animals must be able to live with the vaccine.

181. Heneson, Nancy and Christopher Joyce. "AIDS: A Suitable Place for Treatment?" New Scientist, v. 109, March 13, 1986, p. 24.

Researchers have singled out the TAT, or trans-activating gene, as a potential target for stopping the AIDS virus. By knocking out this gene, the virus will be unable to reproduce.

182. "Investigators Study AIDS Epidemiology and Drug Treatment." American Family Physician, v. 32, December 1985, p. 206.

Recent studies indicate that the drug suramin can stop the AIDS virus from reproducing. However, none of the patients in the test showed any clinical improvement. The search is under way for an antiviral agent to combat AIDS.

183. "Isoprinosine Unproven." FDA Consumer, v. 19, September 1985, pp. 37-38.

There is no evidence that isoprinosine can help combat AIDS. It is not approved by the FDA for any medical purpose despite the fact that the manufacturer claims that it helps stimulate the immune system.

184. Klatzmann, David and Luc Montagnier. "Approaches to AIDS Therapy." Nature, v. 319, January 2, 1986, pp. 10-11.

The development of an immunosuppressant drug (cyclosporin-a) to treat AIDS has received a great deal of publicity. Three rational approaches to treating AIDS are: 1. Develop drugs that will stop the virus from spreading, 2. Stimulate or reconstitute the immune system, and 3. Treat AIDS as an autoimmune disease, possibly with immunosuppressive drugs.

185. Krause, Richard M. "Koch's Postulates and the Search for the AIDS Agent." Public Health Reports, May/June 1984, pp. 291-299.

Attitudes about AIDS are compared with attitudes about tuberculosis during the nineteenth century. The initial response was to romanticize the disease, but once it was determined to be infectious and contagious, the victims were shunned by society. By following the postulates of Dr. Robert Koch, we should discover the cause of AIDS.

186. Langone, John. "AIDS: The Quest for a Cure." Discover, v. 6, January 1985, pp. 75-77.

The biggest breakthrough of 1984 was the identification of HTLV-III as the AIDS virus in the United States and the LAV virus in France. The story of the discovery of the virus is presented.

187. Marx, Jean L. "AIDS Drug Shows Promise in Preliminary Clinical Trial." Science, v. 231, March 28, 1986, pp. 1504-1505.

The drug AZT has shown some promise in fighting AIDS. AZT works by attaching itself to the DNA chain and interrupting the life cycle of the virus.

188. Marx, Jean L. "A Surprising Action for the AIDS Virus." Science, v. 231, February 21, 1986, p. 798.

The HTLV-III virus reproduces by increasing the translation of messenger RNA into protein. Agents that inhibit this translation may be able to stop the spread of the virus.

189. "A New Aid in Fighting AIDS?" Newsweek, v. 105, February 18, 1985, p. 85.

A spermicide widely available in contraceptive creams and gels has been found to kill the AIDS virus even in very low concentrations.

190. "New Research Leads to AIDS Vaccine." New Scientist, v. 110, April 17, 1986, p. 17.

Researchers in the United States have succeeded in inserting one of the genes from the AIDS virus into another virus. When the second virus is injected into animals, antibodies to the AIDS virus are produced. This procedure could lead to an AIDS vaccine.

191. Norman, Colin. "AIDS Therapy: New Push for Clinical Trials." Science, v. 230, December 20, 1985, pp. 1355-1358.

While much research is being conducted on a drug therapy for AIDS, some aspects of the virus are not possible to be killed by drug therapy. The life cycle of the virus has many stages that all must be stopped. The best method will be in preventing the virus from reproducing. Some drugs currently under trial are discussed.

192. Norman, Colin. "AIDS Virus Presents Moving Target." Science, v. 230, December 20, 1985, p. 1357.

Many problems exist in the pursuit of an AIDS vaccine. The virus mutates and one variation may not be stopped by a given drug. The victims all have antibodies to the virus, but these are usually ineffective. The virus may be transmitted directly from cell to cell and not just through the bloodstream. There is no good animal model for AIDS and there is a high risk that the virus used in a vaccine will mutate and become pathogenic.

193. Ohlendorf, Pat. "Breakthrough Against a Modern Plague." Macleans, v. 98, February 4, 1985, pp. 47-48.

The decoding of the genetic code of the AIDS virus may be the first step in finding a cure. Once the gene sequence is known, it may be possible to genetically engineer a vaccine for the virus.

194. Ohlendorf, Pat. "The Pursuit of a Cure." Macleans, v. 98, August 12, 1985, pp. 36-37.

Although several drugs such as HPA-23 and suramin are being tested on AIDS patients, no cure is in sight. Most attempts to stop AIDS concentrate on building up the patient's immune system, but some scientists believe that we should concentrate on the secondary infections as well.

195. "Research Outlook: Taking All Bets." Hospitals, v. 60, January 5, 1986, p. 59.

Some researchers feel that a treatment for AIDS will be available in two years, but others are not as hopeful. Any drug that will be used to treat AIDS must both inhibit the spread of the virus and boost the patient's immune system.

196. "Researchers Tackle AIDS." High Technology, v. 5, May 1985, p. 8.

Two possible treatments for AIDS have been found. The first is a molecule that stimulates the action of the T-4 cells and the second involves a mineral compound that inhibits the reproduction of the virus.

197. "Retrovaccine." <u>Scientific American</u>, v. 253, August 1985, p. 62.
   A vaccine used for cats to prevent feline leukemia virus may lead to a vaccine for AIDS. The cat virus is a retrovirus similar to HTLV-III.

198. Riesenberg, Donald E. and Charles Marwick. "Anti-AIDS Agents Show Varying Early Results In Vitro and In Vivo." <u>JAMA: Journal of the American Medical Association</u>, **v. 254, November 8, 1985, pp. 2521+.**
   Several experimental drugs have shown some success in combatting AIDS. However, while some look promising, none is yet beyond the trial stage. Several different drugs are highlighted.

199. Silberner, Joanne. "AIDS Announcement Raises Questions." <u>Science News</u>, v. 128, November 9, 1985, p. 293.
   French scientists have announced that the drug cyclosporine works well against AIDS and will begin clinical trials. Scientists in the United States are concerned about the short time period in which the drug was developed and tested.

200. Silberner, Joanne. "AIDS Research, Virus Both Advance." <u>Science News</u>, v. 127, January 5, 1985, p. 7.
   The drug ribavirin has been shown to inhibit the reproduction of the LAV virus. However, before this drug can be clinically tested, the virus seems to be expanding beyond the initial high risk groups.

201. Silberner, Joanne. "AIDS: Waiting for Cure or Treatment." <u>Science News</u>, v. 128, October 12, 1985, p. 229.
   A new drug, azidothymidine, may be used to counteract the AIDS virus. It has shown signs of working against the virus in the test tube and is now being tested on humans.

202. Silberner, Joanne. "Complexing AIDS." <u>Science News</u>, v. 128, October 26, 1985, p. 267.
   AIDS victims with anemia can be helped by transfusions of packed red blood cells. These cells bind to the immune complexes in the blood and take them to the liver to expel them from the body.

203. Silberner, Joanne. "On the AIDS Trail: Work Continues on Test, Cure, Vaccine." <u>Science News</u>, v. 127, February 16, 1985, p. 100.
   One of the obstacles to an AIDS vaccine is that the virus changes frequently. A new blood test currently under development may be more accurate than the test now in use and the antiviral drug HPA-23 has shown some success in fighting AIDS.

204. Siwolop, Sana. "AIDS Drugs: Some Relief, But Adverse Side Effects." Discover, v. 6, December 1985, p. 38.

A cure for AIDS will not be available for at least five years. However, a number of drugs are being tested to determine their effectiveness in relieving the symptoms of AIDS. Some of these drugs are profiled.

205. "Suramin Drug Is Disappointing in AIDS." New Scientist, v. 107, September 26, 1985, p. 30.

Suramin, a drug used to treat African trypanosomiasis and onchocerciasis, did not help in treating AIDS. Of ten patients treated, none showed any improvement. Of six patients with Kaposi's sarcoma, two actually showed enlarged sarcomas at the end of the trial.

206. Teitelman, Robert. "The Promise of AIDS." Forbes, v. 134, November 19, 1985, pp. 302+.

While no AIDS cure has been found, researchers have discovered that the agent causing AIDS is the HTLV-III virus. This virus kills the helper T-cells, shutting down the immune system. Some genetic engineering companies are working on solutions to the AIDS problem.

207. Ticer, Scott. "Fast-Buck Artists Are Making a Killing on AIDS." Business Week, December 2, 1985, pp. 85-86.

Many AIDS victims are travelling abroad to buy experimental drugs or are buying cures in this country that are sold by con-artists. There is no evidence that any of these drugs have any effect on AIDS.

208. "Two Steps Closer to Stopping AIDS." Science Digest, v. 93, April 1985, p. 19.

Two breakthroughs in AIDS research have been the development of a blood test that identifies antibodies to the AIDS virus and the discovery that the drug suramin inhibits the reproduction of the virus.

209. Walgate, Robert. "Politics of Premature French Claim of Cure." Nature, v. 318, November 7, 1985, p. 3.

The French claim to a cure for AIDS, cyclosporine, was made prematurely due to pressure by the French government. The drug will soon undergo clinical trials, but it appears to work by blocking the action of mature T-4 cells and causing the body to produce new ones.

210. Wallis, Claudia. "Furor Over an AIDS Announcement." Time, v. 126, November 11, 1985, p. 77.

French scientists have announced that they are testing cyclosporin on AIDS patients. American researchers do not believe that enough background research has been done to show that the drug will be safe and effective.

211. Weber, Jonathon. "AIDS: The Virus Is Not Immune." New Scientist, v. 109, January 2, 1986, pp. 37-39.

Several drugs are currently being tested for their use in fighting AIDS. These drugs act by inhibiting the reproduction of the virus at various stages or by boosting the immune response. Cyclosporin A, suramin, HPA-23, isoprinosine, and several other drugs are featured.

212. "Where Now With AIDS?" Nature, v. 313, January 24, 1985, p. 254.

The publication of the complete nucleotide sequence of the AIDS virus will help to better characterize the disease. It is possible that these sequences will help those researchers working on a vaccine to find a cure for AIDS soon before the number of victims rises dramatically.

213. Wright, Karen. "AIDS Protein Made." Nature, v. 319, February 13, 1986, p. 525.

A part of the AIDS virus has been genetically engineered by an American company and a protein from the AIDS virus has been implanted in another virus with favorable results. This procedure may lead to an AIDS vaccine.

214. Wright, Karen. "State Aid Offered for Vaccine." Nature, v. 321, May 8, 1986, p. 105.

Legislation eliminating product liability for an AIDS vaccine is being pushed through the California legislature. It is hoped that this will remove one of the economic obstacles to vaccine development.

215. Young, Lowell S. "Management of Opportunistic Infection Complicating the Acquired Immunodeficiency Syndrome." Medical Clinics of North America, v. 70, May 1986, pp. 677-692.

There is no clinical evidence that any treatments for AIDS will prolong the life of the patient. While many researchers are developing drugs to treat the secondary infections, the highest priority should be to find an agent that kills the AIDS virus.

AIDS Hysteria, Fears, and Fallacies

216. Adler, Jerry et al. "The AIDS Conflict." <u>Newsweek</u>, v. 106, September 23, 1985, pp. 18-24.

The ethical and social implications of AIDS may be far more damaging than the disease itself. Children are being kept out of school, blood donations are down, and groups are promoting safer methods of sexual activity. Many anti-gay groups are using AIDS to increase their activities against the gay community.

217. "AIDS Hunt: Precaution or Privacy Violation?" <u>Newsweek</u>, v. 106, September 2, 1985, p. 27.

The state of Colorado is requiring that doctors and laboratories report the names of all persons testing positive for the AIDS virus. Many people feel that this is a violation of privacy rights.

218. "AIDS, Nature, and the Nature of AIDS." <u>National Review</u>, v. 37, November 1, 1985, p. 18.

The story of AIDS is concentrating on sympathy for the victims and does not emphasize the sexual promiscuity that led to the disease. It is the gay lifestyle itself that brought about the spread of AIDS.

219. Allen, Glen. "Ethics and AIDS." <u>World Press Review</u>, v. 33, February 1986, p. 53.

The AIDS crisis creates an ethical problem for public health officials. The health of the community must be measured against the rights of the individual. The only weapon available right now is public education about the disease.

220. Allen, Glen. "The Ethics of AIDS." <u>Macleans</u>, v. 98, November 18, 1985, pp. 2+.

The issues of confidentiality and public health are conflicting in the case of AIDS. Some health and government officials advocate reporting and even isolating victims, whereas others are against those policies. Some positive aspects of the crisis are that victims and potential victims are taking the necessary steps to halt the spread of AIDS.

221. Alter, Jonathan. "Sins of Omission." <u>Newsweek</u>, v. 106, September 23, 1985, p. 25.

An evaluation of the press coverage of the AIDS story. In most cases the press has acted responsibly, with the exception of not being specific enough about the exact methods of transmission of the virus.

222. Amiel, Barbara. "AIDS and the Rights of the Well." <u>Macleans</u>, v. 98, September 30, 1985, p. 11.

By keeping the identity of AIDS victims secret, we are exposing the rest of society to the disease. The political protection of homosexuality is endangering the rest of society. We must identify and isolate AIDS victims in order to protect the public at large.

223. "The Backlash Builds Against AIDS." <u>U.S. News and World Report</u>, v. 99, November 4, 1985, p. 9.

Due to a fear of AIDS, many organizations are beginning to take action. The military is screening for AIDS and New York State is closing gay bathhouses. Gay leaders fear retribution and persecution as the disease spreads.

224. Barber, John. "An Epidemic of Fear." <u>Macleans</u>, v. 98, September 23, 1985, pp. 61-63.

Many parents are withholding their children from attending school with AIDS victims. While there is no risk of contracting the disease and experts are trying to educate the public, fear of AIDS is causing many people to act irresponsibly and avoid AIDS victims.

225. Barnes, Fred. "The Politics of AIDS." <u>New Republic</u>, v. 193, November 4, 1985, pp. 11-14.

AIDS has become a rallying point for right wing politicians. Some want to isolate victims and others want to close bathhouses and gay bars. Hopefully, fear of AIDS will not be used to stir up the hatred of homosexuals.

226. Bayer, Ronald. "AIDS and the Gay Community: Between the Specter and the Promise of Medicine." <u>Social Research</u>, **v. 52, Autumn 1985, pp. 581-606.**

The response to AIDS by the public has been one of both subtle and flagrant homophobia. Some see AIDS as the wrath of God or want victims quarantined. Just as gays had confronted the medical establishment and removed homosexuality from the category of diseases, medicine is now forcing the gay community to examine its own behaviors. Medicine has the promise of treating or curing AIDS, but it may also be used by the state to further persecute gay men.

227. Black, David and Edmund White. "The Story of the Year." <u>Rolling Stone</u>, December 19, 1985, pp. 121+.

Fear of AIDS has led to a climate of irrationality that confuses the issues. Only when the media and the government stop publicizing the hysteria of AIDS and start publicizing the facts will we be able to responsibly approach the disease.

228. Buckley, William F. "The AIDS Question." National Review, v. 37, October 18, 1985, p. 63.
Society should not differentiate between the different classes of AIDS victims. However, the fears of non-victims are quite rational and we should safeguard the uninfected as much as possible to protect the majority of society.

229. Cecchi, Robert. "Living with AIDS: When the System Fails." American Journal of Nursing, v. 86, January 1986, pp. 45-47.
The traditional health care system does not function well for AIDS victims. AIDS patients often are isolated and neglected. Sometimes funeral directors will even refuse to embalm and bury the bodies of AIDS patients.

230. Check, William. "Public Education on AIDS: Not Only the Media's Responsibility." Hastings Center Report, v. 15, August 1985, supplement pp. 27-31.
Because the media can distort medical information, public health officials need to mount a continuing education effort to keep the public well-informed about AIDS. The social, political, and psychological issues are enormous, but proper education can minimize fears and misconceptions about AIDS.

231. "Damage Control." Time, v. 126, November 4, 1985, p. 25.
Efforts to contain the social cost of AIDS are becoming increasingly widespread. The military and a number of insurance companies are requiring blood tests and some organizations are promoting safer sexual procedures.

232. Franklin, Deborah. "AIDS: Protecting Two Publics." Science 85, v. 6, December 1985, pp. 16-17.
The medical community must protect the public while still observing the civil rights of those affected. While there is no evidence that casual contact will spread AIDS, many businesses and some health care workers are in favor of firing or quarantining anyone testing positive for the virus.

233. Gergen, David R. "What Answers for AIDS?" U.S. News and World Report, v. 99, September 23, 1985, p. 78.
As AIDS spreads, the fear of AIDS is also growing. Millions of Americans are now forced to make decisions related to the disease. A national response is called for and AIDS victims should be quarantined.

234. Goldsmith, Marsha F. "Hastings Center Initiates AIDS Study." JAMA: Journal of the American Medical Association, v. 254, November 8, 1985, p. 2527.
The Hastings Center is initiating a study on the social and ethical implications of AIDS. Appropriate uses of the AIDS blood test will be the first factor studied.

235. Harrison, Barbara G. "It's Okay to Be Angry About AIDS." Mademoiselle, v. 92, February 1986, p. 96.

There is no clear concensus on AIDS except for the fear of the disease. The AIDS crisis may bring out the worst in us all and we should all look for the best response within ourselves.

236. Heneson, Nancy. "AIDS: A Public Health Disaster." New Scientist, v. 108, November 14, 1985, pp. 75-76.

The public health aspects of AIDS are extremely complex. The most prominent problem is the conflict between the rights of the individual and the welfare of the public. Efforts to make the bathhouse environment safer or to test the blood of military recruits can be seen as either medical or political decisions.

237. "In Pursuit of AIDS." New Scientist, v. 105, February 7, 1985, p. 2.

At a time when millions of people are suffering from diseases commonly associated with poverty, medical researchers are concentrating on a disease which affects relatively few people, AIDS. The medical establishment and journals should evaluate information about AIDS and not get carried away by the newness of the disease.

238. Klass, Perri. "What Should a Doctor Tell a Patient?" Discover, v. 6, October 1985, pp. 20-21.

Fear of AIDS may lead patients to greatly exaggerate possible symptoms in their minds. Doctors should not mention that a patient could possibly have AIDS until test results have been received.

239. Lunsden, Andrew. "J'Accuse." New Statesman, v. 110, July 19, 1985, p. 25.

The British media has been highly prejudicial towards gays when dealing with the AIDS issue. It has sensationalized, moralized, and spread much more misinformation than either its American or European counterparts.

240. Mano, D. Keith. "The Politicization of AIDS." National Review, v. 38, February 28, 1986, pp. 59-60.

Many liberals are blaming political decisions for the AIDS crisis and conservatives feel that it is a deserved repercussion of gay immorality. Although the disease is frightening and irreversible, gays who practice promiscuous sex are bringing the disease upon themselves.

241. Marwick, Charles. "Information, Consideration Needed." <u>JAMA: Journal of the American Medical Association</u>, v. 253, June 21, 1985, pp. 3376-3377.

A number of lessons can be learned from the way government and the medical community have responded to the AIDS crisis. Mandatory reporting of AIDS victims should not be done, the issue of confidentiality has not been dealt with, the system slows a good scientific response to the disease, communication of AIDS information to the public has been poor, and a method of funding medical emergencies needs to be established.

242. Morrow, Lance. "The Start of a Plague Mentality." <u>Time</u>, v. 126, September 23, 1985, p. 92.

Fear of AIDS is bringing about a plague mentality with respect to homosexuals. Some feel that AIDS is a punishment for sin and others react to it as a conflict between order and chaos. As opposed to the bomb, AIDS is a death that lingers and sneaks up unexpectedly on its victims.

243. "The New AIDS Risk: A Term in Jail." <u>Newsweek</u>, v. 106, October 28, 1985, p. 98.

The city of San Antonio has made it a crime for an AIDS victim to have sex with a healthy person or for AIDS to be spread through other means.

244. "No AIDS for Britain's Peers." <u>Discover</u>, v. 6, May 1985, p. 8.

Burke's Peerage, the social register of the British aristocracy, has decided not to list anyone who has AIDS.

245. "A Plague on Homosexuals?" <u>Economist</u>, v. 294, March 2, 1985, pp. 16-17.

Most people have no chance of contracting AIDS, but a great fear of the disease has overtaken society. We must all learn the true medical facts about AIDS and avoid misinformation if we are to effectively fight this disease.

246. Press, Aric, Susan Agrest, and Daniel Pedersen. "AIDS and Civil Rights." <u>Newsweek</u>, v. 106, November 18, 1985, pp. 86-89.

The New York City government has closed one bathhouse because it was afraid of the spread of AIDS. This and other legal actions are being seen by gay rights groups as an attempt to limit the civil rights of homosexuals.

247. Relman, Arnold S. **"AIDS: The Emerging Ethical Dilemmas."** <u>Hastings Center Report</u>, v. 15, August 1985, supplement pp. 1-12.

AIDS was discovered in 1981 when physicians began reporting cases of unusual infections in young homosexual men. It was soon determined that the disease is communicable and is now spreading quickly. There is no hope for an immediate cure, despite the vast amounts of research currently underway.

248. Serrill, Michael S. "A Scourge Spreads Panic." Time, v. 126, October 28, 1985, pp. 50-52.

AIDS has spread to fifty countries and is becoming a world-wide problem. Members of high risk groups in many nations are suffering from discrimination because of fear of the disease.

249. "Should AIDS Victims Be Isolated?" U.S. News and World Report, v. 99, September 30, 1985, p. 50.

Some politicians and medical researchers have advocated the quarantining of AIDS patients until a cure is found. The pros and cons of isolation are debated.

250. Silverman, Mervyn F. and Deborah B. Silverman. "AIDS and the Threat to Public Health." Hastings Center Report, v. 15, August 1985, supplement pp. 19-22.

AIDS has raised many ethical questions for the public health community. Sex education efforts must now concentrate on methods for having safe gay sex. Records on AIDS patients must be kept confidential, but an individual patient has the right to know about his/her condition. Social and political decisions weighing the need to control the disease against the rights of the individuals must be made.

251. Sobran, Joseph. "The Politics of AIDS." National Review, v. 38, May 23, 1986, pp. 22-26+.

Fighting AIDS should be a purely medical problem, but gay activists have manipulated AIDS for their own needs. They squelch any public health provisions that inhibit their lifestyle, requiring the public to pay for gay indulgence.

252. "A Social Disease." Nation, v. 241, September 14, 1985, pp. 195-196.

AIDS is a social disease that is also encased in social, political, and cultural ignorance. When diseases strike less socially acceptable groups, the general public is not interested. It is too bad that it must strike a movie star or businessman before we become involved.

253. "A Special Challenge of AIDS: Providing Facts, Calming Fears." Public Health Reports, v. 99, January/February 1984, pp. 99-100.

Some means of providing information by the Public Health Service about AIDS to the public are highlighted, including meetings and conferences, a national hotline, videotapes, and publications.

254. Stein, M. L. "AIDS: Getting the Facts." Editor and Publisher, v. 118, November 2, 1985, pp. 16-17.

The news media tends to emphasize the negative aspects of AIDS and hurts the public education efforts. Journalists should seek out knowledgeable medical advisors to help with their stories.

255. Svesko, Vladimir. "AIDS in the Emergency Room." New York, v. 18, September 23, 1985, pp. 36-37.

AIDS patients who come to the emergency room of a New York hospital are subjected to substandard facilities and inadequate treatment. Often they are just sent home and told to see a private physician or an AIDS clinic.

256. Tancredi, Laurence R. and Nora D. Volkow. "AIDS: Its Symbolism and Ethical Considerations." Medical Heritage, v. 2, January/February 1986, pp. 12-18.

Many people are associating the AIDS crisis with the sins of homosexuals and see the disease as revenge for immorality. Researchers and health care workers dealing with AIDS must set aside any individual and societal values and look only at the medical facts of AIDS in order to deal with the disease in a rational manner.

257. Thomas, Evan. "The New Untouchables." Time, v. 126, September 23, 1985, pp. 24-26.

Fear of AIDS is reaching epidemic proportions. This fear is far out of proportion in contrast to the actual risk of contracting the disease. Gay rights groups are trying to differentiate between the actual risks and the hysteria.

258. Trafford, Abigail et al. "The Politics of AIDS: A Tale of Two States." U.S. News and World Report, v. 99, November 18, 1985, pp. 70-71.

In Texas, a state among the top five in number of AIDS cases, the health commissioner proposed that AIDS patients be quarantined. The conservatism of the state is making a response to AIDS slow to achieve. In Montana, with one reported case, the response has been one of curiosity.

259. "What Nurses Think About Gay AIDS Victims." RN, v. 48, July 1985, pp. 10-11.

In a homophobia test given to nurses and physicians at a New York City hospital, the women nurses were found to have a much more negative attitude than the male physicians. It is theorized that the nurses are more afraid of AIDS patients because they deal with the patients on a much more frequent basis than the physicians.

Case Studies of AIDS Victims

260. Allan, Gene et al. "The New Terror of AIDS." Macleans, v. 98, August 12, 1985, pp. 32-35.

AIDS is a terrifying disease with no known cure that always leads to the death of its victims. Five Canadian AIDS patients are profiled and the medical, psychological, and social effects of the disease are examined.

261. Blackwell, Marie. "AIDS In the Family." Essence, v. 16, August 1985, pp. 54-56+.

The story of how one woman's family reacted when they learned that her thirty-six year old brother had AIDS. Without the support of family, his experience with AIDS would have been much worse.

262. Carlson, Peter and Carole Patton. "AIDS: Fatal, Incurable, and Spreading." People, v. 23, June 17, 1985, pp. 42-49.

The case study of a man who is a hemophiliac and contracted AIDS through blood transfusions. He then passed the disease on to his wife through sexual contact and to their son during pregnancy or through breast milk. He is angry at the medical establishment for not yet finding a cure.

263. Crovella, Alexina C. "The Person Behind the Disease." Nursing 85, v. 15, September 1985, pp. 42-43.

The story of how the staff and patients at an alcohol/drug rehabilitation center reacted when an AIDS patient was admitted for treatment.

264. Ferrera, Anthony J. "My Personal Experience with AIDS." American Psychologist, v. 39, November 1984, pp. 1285-1287.

A chronicle of how one man dealt with AIDS from the initial diagnosis to his death. His friends and the hospital staff were very supportive and helped him cope with the disease.

265. Greene, Johnny. "A Writer Fights a Faceless Enemy and Learns to Live with Fear." People, v. 23, June 17, 1985, pp. 48-49.

A narrative of how one AIDS victim lives with the disease. He has fought AIDS for one year and now sees hope in experimental new treatments.

266. Haller, Scot. "AIDS in the Family." People, v. 24, November 18, 1985, pp. 136-142.

The story of how one man and his family have dealt with AIDS.

267. Morrisroe, Patricia. "AIDS: One Man's Story." New York, v. 18, August 19, 1985, pp. 28-35.

A personal narrative of how one man is coping with AIDS. While many of his friends have already died, he is fighting against all odds to beat the disease.

268. Peabody, Barbara. "Living with AIDS: A Mother's Perspective." American Journal of Nursing, v. 86, January 1986, pp. 45-46.

A mother provides a personal narrative on how AIDS led to the death of her son. As a nurse and a mother, she showed a great deal of support and kept his hopes high.

269. Seligmann, Jean and Nikki F. Greenberg. "Only Months to Live and No Place to Die." Newsweek, v. 106, August 12, 1985, p. 26.

An AIDS patient with only six months to live has been rejected by hospitals, hospices, and his former friends. He drifted through life with no place to die until his cause was picked up in a local newspaper story and some volunteers came forward to offer him shelter.

270. Seligmann, Jean and Michael Reese. "A Family Gives Refuge to a Son Who Has AIDS." Newsweek, v. 106, August 12, 1985, p. 24.

The story of how one man's family reacted when they found out that he had AIDS. Rather than running away, they have provided him with a caring and loving environment.

271. Spechko, Phyllis L. "Knowing Ron." JAMA: Journal of the American Medical Association, v. 253, February 15, 1985, p. 985.

A personal narrative on how AIDS affected one patient. Ron was slowly drained of his energy and health while he fought to remain active, independent, and lovable.

AIDS and Health Care Workers

272. "AIDS Anxiety." <u>Time</u>, v. 124, December 24, 1984, p. 59.
   A medical technician with AIDS insisted that he contracted the disease by pricking himself with a needle used to take blood samples and in another case a nurse became ill after injecting herself with blood from an AIDS patient. However, there is very little risk that other health care workers can contract the disease.

273. "Health Personnel May Have Gotten AIDS From Patients." <u>RN</u>, v. 48, December 1985, p. 6.
   The cases of two health care workers who claim to have contracted AIDS from needlesticks and cuts are reported. The Centers for Disease Control still maintain that the chances of health care workers catching AIDS are extremely remote.

274. "Is There Risk to Health Care Workers?" <u>American Journal of Nursing</u>, v. 85, September 1985, p. 972.
   The likelihood of AIDS transmission to health care workers is very small. No case of a health care worker contracting AIDS through treating AIDS patients has yet been documented.

275. "Update: Evaluation of Human T-Lymphotropic Virus Type III/Lymphadenopathy Associated Virus Infection in Health-Care Personnel: United States." <u>MMWR: Morbidity and Mortality Weekly Report</u>, v. 34, September 27, 1985, pp. 575-578.
   Two cases of health care workers who possibly contracted AIDS on the job are presented. The first case involves a woman who had sustained needlestick injuries and the second involved a man who sustained an accidental cut while processing blood supplies. There is still very little risk to health care personnel.

276. "Update: Prospective Evaluation of Health-Care Workers Exposed Via the Parenteral or Mucous-Membrane Route to Blood or Body Fluids from Patients with Acquired Immunodeficiency Syndrome: United States." <u>MMWR: Morbidity and Mortality Weekly Report</u>, v. 34, February 22, 1985, pp. 101-103.
   Health care workers who had exposures to blood, saliva, urine, or other bodily fluids of AIDS patients were monitored to determine if there is any risk to such exposure. Of 361 health care workers reporting exposures, none showed antibodies to the AIDS virus. There is very little risk to health care personnel.

277. Volberding, Paul and Donald Abrams. "Clinical Care and Research in AIDS." Hastings Center Report, v. 15, August 1985, supplement pp. 16-18.

Three recommendations are made for physicians when working with AIDS patients: 1. Because AIDS cannot be transmitted by casual contact, no patient should be denied treatment, 2. Identities of AIDS patients should be kept confidential, and 3. AIDS patients should have access to the same high quality care as any other patient.

278. Wachter, Robert M. "The Impact of the Acquired Immunodeficiency Syndrome on Medical Residency Training." New England Journal of Medicine, v. 314, January 16, 1986, pp. 177-180.

Physicians undergoing residency requirements in urban areas are exposed to a disproportionate number of AIDS cases during their training. There is very little risk of the physician contracting the disease. Recommendations are given for working with AIDS patients.

279. Weiss, Stanley H. et al. "HTLV-III Infection Among Health Care Workers." JAMA: Journal of the American Medical Association, v. 254, October 18, 1985, pp. 2089-2093.

Health care workers from institutions with a large number of AIDS cases were examined for antibodies to the AIDS virus. The risk of transmission is low, but medical personnel must be trained in the proper handling of instruments used on AIDS patients.

280. "You're Not Likely to Get AIDS From Patients." RN, v. 48, June 1985, pp. 12-13.

In a survey of hospital employees who had worked with AIDS patients, not one person had antibodies to the virus. There is almost no chance of a hospital worker catching AIDS from a patient.

AIDS in Prisons, the Military, and the Workplace

281. Adler, Jerry and Nikki F. Greenberg. "Trying to Lock Out AIDS." Newsweek, v. 106, September 16, 1985, p. 65.

Prison officials and military officers are both concerned about the spread of AIDS within their respective institutions. All military recruits will now face a mandatory AIDS blood test. Gay rights groups claim that this is really a method to exclude gays from military service.

282. "AIDS in the Workplace: An Epidemic of Fear." National Safety and Health News, v. 133, January 1986, pp. 34-39.

AIDS is spreading quickly and will require policy decisions in every large company. Many of the problems related to AIDS are due to misinformation. The disease and its methods of transmission are discussed.

283. "AIDS: No Need for Worry in the Workplace." Newsweek, v. 106, November 25, 1985, p. 51.

There is no evidence that AIDS can be transmitted through casual contact in offices, schools, or factories.

284. Beardsley, Tim. "U.S. Troops and AIDS." Nature, v. 316, August 22, 1985, p. 668.

The Defense Department is going to require civilian blood banks to disclose the names of all active duty military personnel who test positively for the AIDS virus. Blood banks fear that military personnel will refuse to donate blood and gay rights activists fear persecution of gays by the military.

285. Glasbrenner, Kimberly. "Prisons Confront Dilemma of Inmates with AIDS." JAMA: Journal of the American Medical Association, v. 255, May 9, 1986, pp. 2399-2404.

AIDS could become a major health problem for correction facilities due to the close confinement of many men in high risk groups. Some prisons are testing new inmates for antibodies to the virus, but even those persons who are tested positive are not isolated. Many facilities are establishing educational programs for inmates.

286. "Group Health Insurers Do Not Exclude AIDS Cover." Business Insurance, v. 19, September 30, 1985, p. 61.

Group insurance policies do plan to include AIDS patients in their policies. The increased expenses are expected to be picked up by particular high risk policy holders.

287. Halcrow, Allan. "AIDS in the Workplace." Personnel Journal, v. 64, October 1985, pp. 10-11.
There is no evidence that AIDS can be transmitted in the workplace. AIDS can only be spread through intimate contact. Some cities have passed laws forbidding discrimination against AIDS victims and some businesses are taking out insurance policies to cover the costs of employees with AIDS.

288. Hammett, Theodore M. AIDS in Prisons and Jails: Issues and Options. Washington, D.C.: National Institute of Justice, February 1986. 8p. Superintendent of Documents Number J28.24:Ai2.
Since 1981, 455 confirmed cases of AIDS have been found in state and federal prison populations. AIDS poses a real danger to inmates because there are many high risk individuals in close confinement. The medical and legal issues involved in testing for and dealing with AIDS are presented.

289. Hammett, Theodore M. and Monique Sullivan. **AIDS in Correctional Facilities: Issues and Options**. Washington, D.C.: National Institute of Justice, April 1986. 217p. Superintendent of Documents Number J28.28:Ai1.
Over 450 cases of AIDS have been confirmed in correctional facilities in the United States. Prisoners are at risk due to close confinement with members of high risk populations. The policy questions involved in the screening of prisoners for AIDS, educating staff and inmates, and the legal issues of AIDS in prisons are discussed.

290. "Insurers Need Aids Tests, Doctor Says." National Underwriter (Life and Health Insurance Edition), v. 89, October 5, 1985, pp. 4+.
Insurance companies would like to use the AIDS blood test to screen AIDS victims. They claim that it is unfair to other policyholders who will have to pay the cost of AIDS claims.

291. "Keep Insurer AIDS Tests: M.D." National Underwriter (Property and Casualty Insurance Edition), v. 89, October 4, 1985, pp. 3+.
AIDS insurance policies must be careful to comply with statutes of confidentiality of medical records and unfair discrimination. The AIDS blood test is vital to insurance decisions and should be available for company use.

292. Kocolowski, Linda. "Insurers Gear Up to Examine Impact of AIDS." National Underwriter (Life and Health Insurance Edition), v. 89, September 21, 1985, pp. 4+.
Insurance companies are becoming concerned about AIDS. They are tracking AIDS claims and some companies may begin to use the blood test despite state laws against such use. Insurance companies are afraid of losing a large amount of money due to AIDS.

293. Mason, James O. "Statement on the Development of Guidelines for the Prevention of AIDS Transmission in the Workplace." Public Health Reports, v. 101, January/February 1986, pp. 6-8.

The Public Health Service has issued guidelines about AIDS for health care workers, personal service workers, food service workers, and other employees. These guidelines are based on experience with Hepatitis B and are summarized in this article.

294. Norman, Colin. "Military AIDS Testing Offers Research Bonus." Science, v. 232, May 16, 1986, pp. 818-820.

Congress appropriated $40 million to the Army for AIDS research without passing the necessary authorizing legislation. Following individuals who test positive for the antibody to the AIDS virus can produce valuable information about how AIDS is transmitted. Blood testing for AIDS is complicated by the fact that drug use and homosexuality are both grounds for dismissal from the service.

295. Pave, Irene. "Fear and Loathing in the Workplace: What Managers Can Do About AIDS." Business Week, November 25, 1985, p. 126.

Companies are beginning to wonder how to deal with AIDS. Isolation and/or blood tests will do nothing to help the situation. Counseling and education are the best approaches.

296. "Pentagon AIDS Test That Sparked Furor." U.S. News and World Report, v. 99, September 9, 1985, p. 12.

The military has decided to test all recruits for AIDS. Those who test positive will be denied entry into the service. Gay rights leaders believe that it is merely a method to discriminate against homosexuals.

297. "Recommendations for Preventing Transmission of Infection with Human T-Lymphotropic Virus Type III/Lymphadenopathy Associated Virus in the Workplace." MMWR: Morbidity and Mortality Weekly Report, v. 34, November 15, 1985, pp. 681-695.

There is no known risk of contracting AIDS from working with a victim. The only occupation in which AIDS might be a problem is in the health care industry. Guidelines for workers dealing with AIDS victims are provided for health care workers, personal service workers, food service workers, and others working in the same environment as an AIDS victim.

298. Shahoda, Terry, Theresa Lashley, and Janet Firshein. "Insurers: Watchful But Not Worried." Hospitals, v. 60, January 5, 1986, p. 58.

Health insurance companies are keeping a watchful eye on the AIDS crisis, but none have yet changed their policies. As AIDS spreads, insurance companies and state medical plans may have to place AIDS patients in high risk pools.

299. Taravella, Steve. "Alternative Care Helps Firms Reduce Costs to Treat AIDS." <u>Business Insurance</u>, v. 19, September 30, 1985, pp. 1+.

Employers are seeking alternative health care plans to handle AIDS victims. Some companies are also screening prospective employees for exposure to the AIDS virus. AIDS has the potential to bring about very high medical expenses.

300. "Test Insurance Applicants for Signs of AIDS?" <u>U.S. News and World Report</u>, v. 99, November 25, 1985, p. 71.

Many insurance companies are considering requiring AIDS blood tests before issuing a policy. Two insurance executives give the pros and cons of this procedure.

Psychological Aspects of AIDS

301. Abrams, Donald I. et al. "Routine Care and Psychosocial Support of the Patient with the Acquired Immunodeficiency Syndrome." *Medical Clinics of North America*, v. 70, May 1986, pp. 707-720.

Proper care of AIDS patients requires attention to the psychological and sociological problems associated with the disease. Some experiences gained in San Francisco are described.

302. Batchelor, Walter F. "AIDS." *American Psychologist*, v. 39, November 1984, pp. 1277-1278.

The vast majority of AIDS research has focused on epidemiology, disease transmission, causes, and studies of immunology. An overview of the psychological and emotional aspects of AIDS is provided.

303. Batchelor, Walter F. "AIDS: A Public Health and Psychological Emergency." *American Psychologist*, v. 39, November 1984, pp. 1279-1284.

AIDS is a mental health as well as a medical emergency. Data collection, clinical research, and medical practices have suffered from the lack of information on the psychological factors of the disease.

304. Bennett, Dawn D. "Like Sheep Virus, AIDS Virus Infects Brain." *Science News*, v. 127, January 12, 1985, p. 127.

The AIDS virus may attack the brain as well as the immune system. There are definite similarities between a virus that causes neurologic diseases in sheep and the HTLV-III virus.

305. Coates, Thomas J., Lydi Temoshok, and Jeffrey Mandel. "Psychosocial Research Is Essential to Understanding and Treating AIDS." *American Psychologist*, v. 39, November 1984, pp. 1309-1314.

Psychosocial stresses have a significant effect on the functioning of the immune system. Research should draw on epidemiological evidence and examine the role of individuals at risk for AIDS, the role of health professionals, and the lack of cross-cultural and interdisciplinary research needed for a thorough understanding of the disease.

306. "Dementia and AIDS." *American Family Physician*, v. 32, August 1985, pp. 239-242.

Many AIDS patients have mental disorders related to neurological degeneration. CAT scans of AIDS patients resemble those of 80-year-olds rather than 35-year-olds. The mental state of AIDS patients should be constantly monitored.

307. Dilley, James W. et al. "Findings in Psychiatric Consultations with Patients with Acquired Immune Deficiency Syndrome." American Journal of Psychiatry, v. 142, January 1985, pp. 82-86.

Of forty AIDS patients studied in a large city hospital, thirteen needed psychiatric care. Dealing with their illness, social isolation, and guilt over their lifestyle all led to depression. The roles of the primary physician and the mental health professional are discussed.

308. Joseph, Jill G. et al. "Coping with the Threat of AIDS." American Psychologist, v. 39, November 1984, pp. 1297-1302.

A project to provide scientifically valid and community-relevant research on the psycho-social aspects of AIDS is described. The program concentrates on obtaining qualitative data, developing inventories, sampling the community, building community networks, and characterizing the crisis of AIDS.

309. Maddox, John. "Further Anxieties About AIDS." Nature, v. 391, January 2, 1986, p. 9.

New findings indicate that AIDS may also attack the nervous system and that some AIDS victims will succumb to neurological rather than pathological conditions. A strategy for fighting AIDS requires a means of stopping the spread of the disease and then finding a means of preventing infections.

310. Martin, John L. and Carole S. Vance. "Behavioral and Psychosocial Factors in AIDS." American Psychologist, v. 39, November 1984, pp. 1303-1308.

Although there are many hypotheses about the causes of AIDS, no firm evidence is available for evaluating them. Studies are needed that employ reliable, valid, and psychometrically sophisticated measures of behavior.

311. Marwick, Charles. "Neurological Complications Appear Often in AIDS." JAMA: Journal of the American Medical Association, v. 253, June 21, 1985, pp. 3379-3383.

AIDS may affect the nervous system much more seriously than previously suspected. Of 370 patients examined, 178 had significant neurological complications. This may be caused by HTLV-III infection of the central nervous system.

312. Meer, Jeff. "AIDS: The Neurological Connection." Psychology Today, v. 20, January 1986, p. 10.

Depression upon learning of AIDS may mask the neurological complications of the disease. There is evidence that the virus attacks the nervous system and disrupts neurons in the brain. These symptoms have been labeled as AIDS Dementia.

313. Morin, Stephen F. and Walter F. Batchelor. "Responding to the Psychological Crisis of AIDS." Public Health Reports, v. 99, January/February 1984, pp. 4-9.

It is the responsibility of the health and mental health communities to respond to the psychological problems of persons with AIDS and to the needs of their lovers and families. The Shanti Project in San Francisco is highlighted and personal testimonies of AIDS victims are presented.

314. Morin, Stephen F., Kenneth A. Charles, and Alan K. Malyon. "The Psychological Impact of AIDS on Gay Men." American Psychologist, v. 39, November 1984, pp. 1288-1293.

AIDS is taking a tremendous psychological toll on its victims and the rest of the gay community. Methods of psychotherapy and sex therapy must be changed in the light of the AIDS crisis. Many gay men must also face the issue of intimacy for the first time.

315. Norman, M. "Behind the Mental Symptoms of AIDS." Psychology Today, v. 18, December 1984, p. 12.

At least 30% of AIDS patients develop psychiatric disorders caused by undiagnosed brain disease. Symptoms include depression, suicidal tendencies, and paranoia. Many of these victims can be treated.

316. Perry, Samual W. and Susan Tross. "Psychiatric Problems of AIDS Inpatients at the New York Hospital: Preliminary Report." Public Health Reports, v. 99, March/April 1984, pp. 200-205.

Of fifty-two patients with AIDS in a New York hospital, neuropsychiatric complications were found in 82% of the victims. AIDS patients have a heightened risk for psychological problems and these are often undiagnosed during acute illness.

317. Sattaur, Omar. "More Evidence for Brain Disease in AIDS." New Scientist, v. 108, October 10, 1985, p. 26.

Further evidence has been found that the AIDS virus also infects the brain. This type of infection is particularly difficult to treat because most drugs do not penetrate the blood-brain barrier.

318. Shaw, George M. "HTLV-III Infection in Brains of Children and Adults with AIDS Encephalopathy." Science, v. 227, January 11, 1986, pp. 177-181.

Unexplained dementia or encephalopathy occurs frequently in children and adults with AIDS. Brain tissue from fifteen infected persons was examined and the AIDS virus was found in five patients. It is thus possible that the AIDS virus also attacks the brain.

Changes in Sexual Behavior Due to AIDS

319. "AIDS Update (Part II)." <u>Harvard Medical School Health Letter</u>, v. 10, December 1985, pp. 2-4.

Until a vaccine for the AIDS virus is developed, the best way to protect yourself against the disease is to be highly selective in choosing sexual partners and to participate only in safe sexual practices.

320. Bruno, Mary et al. "Campus Sex: New Fears." <u>Newsweek</u>, v. 106, October 28, 1985, pp. 81-82.

The AIDS crisis has created a new concern over sex on college campuses. Many schools have appointed advisory committees to decide on how to deal with AIDS and to promote safe sexual practices.

321. Clarke, Gerald. "In the Middle of a War." <u>Time</u>, v. 126, August 12, 1985, p. 46.

Gay men live in fear of AIDS and it is changing their lives. They no longer engage in promiscuous sex and are using safer methods. Counseling groups have appeared throughout the nation to deal with this problem.

322. Cornish, Edward. "Farewell, Sexual Revolution. Hello, New Victorianism." <u>Futurist</u>, v. 20, January/February 1986, pp. 2+.

The AIDS threat is causing many people to rethink their sexual lifestyles. Both men and women are becoming more cautious about who they have as partners and how they have sex. Some predictions of how this will affect the future are made.

323. Gelman, David et al. "The Social Fallout from an Epidemic." <u>Newsweek</u>, v. 106, August 12, 1985, pp. 28-29.

AIDS is causing many changes in sexual practices throughout the nation. Gay men are becoming less promiscuous and prostitutes are making an effort to have safer sex. AIDS may mean the end of the sexual revolution.

324. Levin, Bob. "Facing a Fatal Disease." <u>Macleans</u>, v. 99, January 6, 1986, pp. 48-49.

In a poll of Canadians about AIDS, almost one-half of the respondents were concerned about catching the disease. There were some correlations between concern and sexual habits, but most respondents had made no changes in their lifestyles.

325. Lundberg, George D. "The Age of AIDS: A Great Time for Defensive Living." JAMA: Journal of the American Medical Association, v. 253, June 21, 1985, pp. 3440-3441.

The only way to really lower the risk of contracting AIDS is to change your lifestyle. We must not inject the blood of AIDS patients into others, needles should not be shared, persons with AIDS should not become pregnant, no sexual activity should take place with an AIDS victim, and we should consider testing for AIDS before issuing a marriage license.

326. McKusick, Leon, William Horstman, and Thomas J. Coates. "AIDS and Sexual Behavior Reported by Gay Men in San Francisco." American Journal of Public Health, v. 75, May 1985, pp. 493-496.

Two groups of homosexual men were surveyed about their sexual experiences, one group of men with high risk behavior and one group with fewer sexual partners. Those in the high risk group generally had no change in sexual behavior, but those in the lower risk group showed a substantial reduction in casual sexual contacts.

327. McKusick, Leon et al. "Reported Changes in the Sexual Behavior of Men at Risk for AIDS, San Francisco, 1982-1984: The AIDS Behavioral Research Project." Public Health Reports, v. 100, November/December 1985, pp. 622-629.

Of 454 homosexual men surveyed, a substantial number have reported changes in their sexual behavior. The number of partners and number of times engaging in certain sexual practices declined while the usage of condoms increased.

328. Riesenberg, Donald E. "AIDS-Prompted Behavior Changes Reported." JAMA: Journal of the American Medical Association, v. 255, January 10, 1986, pp. 171-176.

The threat of AIDS is beginning to cause changes in sexual behavior. Homosexual men are reporting a decrease in the number of partners and an increase in safe sexual practices.

329. Schulte, Lucy. "The New Dating Game." New York, v. 19, March 3, 1986, pp. 92-106.

Fear of AIDS is changing the sexual habits of heterosexuals as well as homosexuals. Although the chances of contracting the disease from a single heterosexual contact are slim, many people are using condoms or avoiding sexual encounters altogether.

330. "Self-Reported Behavioral Change Among Gay and Bisexual Men: San Francisco." MMWR: Morbidity and Mortality Weekly Report, v. 34, October 11, 1985, pp. 613-615.

A survey of gay men at risk for AIDS in San Francisco was taken to determine if fear of AIDS has led to any changes in sexual practices. It was found that the average number of sexual partners has decreased and that more men are now engaging in monogamous relationships.

331. Seligmann, Jean et al. "A Nasty New Epidemic." <u>Newsweek</u>, v. 105, February 4, 1985, pp. 72-73.
   The spread of AIDS has caused many Americans to worry about contracting any type of sexually transmitted disease. These diseases can cause infertility or damage a fetus. The risk in cases of sexually transmitted diseases of all types may force us to reassess our sexual lifestyles.

The Legal Problems of AIDS

332. Gest, Ted. "AIDS Triggers Painful Legal Battles." U.S. News and World Report, v. 100, March 24, 1986, pp. 73-74.

Many AIDS victims are using the legal system to fight perceived persecution by employers, schools, and insurance companies. Blood recipients are suing the donating agencies over AIDS. Lawsuits relating to AIDS may soon be flooding the court system.

333. Hyatt, Joshua. "AIDS Is Now Becoming a Legal Epidemic, Too." Inc., v. 7, December 1985, pp. 19-20.

Some AIDS victims are filing lawsuits over employment discrimination. The number of AIDS-related legal cases is expected to rise rapidly.

334. Miller, Patti J. et al. "Potential Liability for Transfusion-Associated AIDS." JAMA: Journal of the American Medical Association, v. 253, June 21, 1985, pp. 3419-3424.

Hospitals, blood banks, and individual physicians may all be legally liable if a patient contracts AIDS through a blood transfusion. Steps should be taken to reduce this risk. If all possible safety factors are followed, the institution and the physician can not be found negligent.

335. Press, Aric. "AIDS Spreads to the Courts." Newsweek, v. 106, July 1, 1985, p. 61.

A woman who contracted AIDS during a blood transfusion has sued her doctor and the blood bank involved. AIDS cases of all types are beginning to flood the judicial system.

336. "Should Nurses Be Told If a Patient Has AIDS?" RN, v. 48, November 1985, p. 10.

A nurse who accidentally stabbed herself with a used hypodermic needle is suing the hospital for not informing her that she was giving injections to an AIDS patient.

AIDS and the Schools

337. "AFRAIDS." New Republic, v. 193, October 14, 1985, pp. 7-10.
The AIDS epidemic has spawned an epidemic of fear throughout the country. This is particularly evident in the movement to keep children with AIDS out of school. There is no evidence that AIDS can be spread through casual contact and no one should be barred from school or work because they have AIDS.

338. "As AIDS Spooks the Schoolroom..." U.S. News and World Report, v. 99, September 23, 1985, p. 7.
New York children boycotted school when an AIDS-infected child was allowed to attend. Despite evidence that AIDS cannot be spread by casual contact, some parents do not wish to risk the health of their children by close contact with an AIDS victim.

339. Conant, Jennet. "AIDS in the Classroom." Newsweek, v. 107, March 3, 1986, p. 6.
A child who was kept out of school because he had AIDS was again barred from school even after health care workers said he could return. A judge ruled that he could not attend because he is carrying a communicable disease.

340. "Education and Foster Care of Children Infected with Human T-Lymphotropic Virus Type III/Lymphadenopathy Associated Virus." MMWR: Morbidity and Mortality Weekly Report, v. 34, August 30, 1985, pp. 517-521.
Almost two hundred cases of AIDS in children under eighteen years of age have been reported. Although there has been a great deal of concern by parents, there has not been a single documented case of any child contracting AIDS at school. Some guidelines are provided for educational and day care institutions that must deal with AIDS victims.

341. "Guidelines for Enrolling Children with AIDS Set Up in Two States." Phi Delta Kappan, v. 66, February 1985, pp. 448-449.
The states of Connecticut and Florida have established official guidelines for the admission of children with AIDS to the public schools. The guidelines urge that the privacy of the children be protected and emphasize that the risk of infection to other children is minimal.

342. McGrath, Ellie. "The AIDS Issue Hits the Schools." Time, v. 126, September 9, 1985, p. 61.
A seventh grade hemophiliac who has contracted AIDS is being kept out of school in Kokomo, Indiana. Although there is no law requiring that he be omitted from public schooling, the superintendent will not allow him in class in order to protect the other students from AIDS.

343. "New Federal Guidelines Say Children with AIDS Can Attend School." Phi Delta Kappan, v. 67, November 1985, pp. 242-244.

Children with AIDS should be allowed to attend school. There is no evidence that normal contact will spread the AIDS virus. Only those children with open wounds or violent behavior should be kept at home.

344. Reed, Sally. "AIDS in the Schools: A Special Report." Phi Delta Kappan**, v. 67, March 1986, pp. 494-498.**

Some school districts are barring children with AIDS from school whereas others are letting the students into regular classes. The medical recommendation is that AIDS is not communicable through casual contact and that there is no danger to other children in a class with an AIDS victim. Employees with AIDS are another problem that school districts must face.

AIDS and the Church

345. "Addressing the AIDS Threat." <u>Christianity Today</u>, v. 29, November 22, 1985, p. 52.

An interview with U.S. Surgeon General C. Everett Koop. In the case of AIDS, the public health reactions coincide with the moral position of a large segment of society. Churches will have problems administering to people who have contracted a deadly disease through sinful behavior.

346. "AIDS: A Christian Response." <u>America</u>, v. 153, August 17, 1985, p. 77.

The Christian community must follow the example of the past and minister to the sick and dying. AIDS should not be treated as retribution for sins against God. To shun an AIDS victim is to shun Christ.

347. Nieckarz, Jim. "Our Fragile Brothers." <u>Commonweal</u>, v. 112, July 12, 1985, pp. 404-406.

A priest learned about AIDS through the death of one of his friends. He then began ministering to AIDS patients and became deeply aware of the fear surrounding the disease. The AIDS crisis challenges us to be good Christians and to set aside our prejudices in order to help those in need.

348. Sattaur, Omar. "Faith, Hope and Bigotry." <u>New Scientist</u>, v. 106, May 16, 1985, p. 45.

AIDS is being used to feed prejudices based on race, sexual preference, or drug abuse. Many religious leaders see AIDS as the wrath of God upon the unholy. These same people ignore other diseases and symptoms that affect only one segment of society.

349. Shelp, Earl E. and Ronald H. Sunderland. "AIDS and the Church." <u>Christian Century</u>, **v. 102, September 11, 1985, pp. 797-800.**

The church has remained silent about AIDS, implying that the victims deserve the disease. Jesus always emphasized compassion for the poor and dispossessed, and his ministry should also apply to AIDS victims. The church should take a leading role in helping AIDS patients.

350. Vaux, Kenneth. "AIDS As Crisis and Opportunity." <u>Christian Century</u>, v. 102, October 16, 1985, pp. 910-911.

AIDS is a medical, political, and religious crisis. The church must ensure that victims receive proper treatment, that the community honors the rights of the victims, and that their congregations are educated about the disease.

AIDS Research, Funding, and Economic Impact

351. Beardsley, Tim. "More for Research and Treatment." Nature, v. 317, October 10, 1985, p. 466.

Congress has added $70 million to the administration's proposed AIDS research budget, bringing the total to $189.7 million. The distribution of these funds to various government agencies is detailed.

352. Beardsley, Tim. "More U.S. Funds for AIDS." Nature, v. 316, August 1, 1985, p. 384.

The Department of Health and Human Services has responded to congressional pressure by allocating an additional $41 million for AIDS research. Some of the new studies that this money will fund are detailed.

353. Brandt, Edward N., Jr. "AIDS Research: Charting New Directions." Public Health Reports, v. 99, September/October 1984, pp. 433-435.

The most important development in AIDS research has been the discovery of the HTLV-III virus. Priorities for the future include: epidemiological studies to determine the natural history of AIDS, evaluation of the AIDS blood test, development of a vaccine, and studies of therapeutic intervention.

354. Budiansky, Stephen. "U.S. Administration's Parsimony Criticized." Nature, v. 313, February 28, 1985, p. 725.

A report from the Office of Technology Assessment is critical of the Reagan Administration's support for AIDS research. The funding levels for AIDS have consistently fallen below necessary levels.

355. Burda, David and Suzanne Powills. "AIDS: A Time Bomb at Hospitals' Door." Hospitals, v. 60, January 5, 1986, pp. 54-61.

AIDS may have a tremendous economic impact on the nation's hospitals. Current costs average $830 per day and insurance companies will not cover all of the costs. Other issues that are raised for hospitals are the isolation of AIDS patients, the transmission of AIDS to health care staff, and the screening of blood.

356. Hardy, Ann M. et al. "The Economic Impact of the First 10,000 Cases of Acquired Immunodeficiency Syndrome in the United States." JAMA: Journal of the American Medical Association, v. 255, January 10, 1986, pp. 209-211.

Expenditures for hospitalization and economic losses from disability have been estimated for the first 10,000 reported cases of AIDS. These patients will require 1.6 million days in the hospital and over $1.4 billion in expenditures. Losses from disabilities and premature death will amount to over $4.8 billion.

357. Holden, Constance. "OTA Critical of AIDS Initiative." Science, v. 227, March 8, 1985, pp. 1182-1183.

The Public Health Service has been underfunded in its fight against AIDS. A recent Office of Technology Assessment report finds that the Public Health Service needs a clear directive and more funds for AIDS research.

358. King, Stephen H. "What State Officials Should Know About AIDS." State Government News, v. 28, September 1985, pp. 8-10.

AIDS is a deadly disease that destroys the immune system and is spread through sexual contact, drug use, or blood transfusions. Many questions related to AIDS will be raised and state governments must respond appropriately.

359. "New AIDS Forecast: A Long, Long Siege." U.S. News and World Report, v. 99, October 14, 1985, p. 14.

The Public Health Service is settling in for a long fight against AIDS, perhaps fifteen years or more. Public information is currently the only mechanism to prevent infection.

360. Norman, Colin. "An Avalanche of New Cash." Science, v. 230, December 29, 1985, p. 1358.

There will be over $240 million spent on AIDS during 1986, double the amount of 1985. Each agency requesting funding received the amount that it wanted.

361. Norman, Colin. "Congress Likely to Halt Shrinkage in AIDS Funds." Science, v. 231, March 21, 1986, pp. 1364-1365.

Although Congress approved $234 million for AIDS research in 1986, that amount has been steadily reduced. Despite the impact of Gramm-Rudman, Congress will work to help keep AIDS funds.

362. Norman, Colin. "Congress Readies AIDS Funding Transfusion." Science, v. 230, October 25, 1985, pp. 418-419.

Prospects for a cure for AIDS do not look good before 1990. The government has made AIDS its number one health priority but is hampered by budget cutbacks. Several different AIDS funding bills are currently working their way through Congress. The primary research areas will be for public education, vaccine development, and drug testing.

363. Norman, Colin. "Institute of Medicine Launches Assessment of AIDS." Science, v. 231, March 28, 1986, p. 1500.

The National Academy of Sciences has begun an assessment of strategies to combat AIDS. The panel will look at both scientific research efforts and public policy associated with AIDS.

364. Palca, Joseph. "Academy Looks for Strategy." Nature, v. 319, February 6, 1986, p. 441.

The National Academy of Science and the Institute of Medicine are attempting to develop a national agenda on research and health care for AIDS. The panel will examine scientific research efforts and the social and public policy issues associated with the disease.

365. Panem, Sandra. "AIDS: Public Policy and Biomedical Research." Hastings Center Report, v. 15, August 1985, supplement pp. 23-26.

Biomedical research is essential in solving the AIDS crisis. However, research priorities in a time of crisis may differ significantly from those during normal periods. Better communication and coordination is needed between the different parts of the health care system if AIDS is going to be stopped.

366. Talbot, David and Larry Bush. "At Risk: While the Reagan Administration Dozes and Scientists Vie for Glory, the Deadly AIDS Epidemic Has Put the Entire Nation At Risk." Mother Jones, v. 10, April 1985, pp. 28-37.

A review of the history of AIDS and the government response. Although the Reagan administration has used AIDS for publicity purposes, it has left AIDS research critically underfunded. The medical establishment is also to blame for its infighting and paranoia.

367. U.S. Congress. House. Committee on Energy and Commerce. Subcommittee on Health and Environment. Acquired Immune Deficiency Syndrome (AIDS). Washington, D.C.: Government Printing Office, 1985. 138p. Superintendent of Documents Number Y4.En2/3:98-185.

The full text of hearings held on September 17, 1984 to examine the state of the AIDS epidemic and AIDS research.

368. U.S. Congress. House. Committee on Government Operations and Committee on Energy and Commerce. Office of Technology Assessment's Findings on the Public Health Service's Response to AIDS. Washington, D.C.: Government Printing Office, 1985. 79p. Superintendent of Documents Number Y4.G74/7:T22/3.

The complete text of a hearing held on February 21, 1985 to assess the government's response to the AIDS crisis.

369. Waldman, Steven. "The Other AIDS Crisis: Who Pays for the Treatment?" Washington Monthly, v. 17, January 1986, pp. 25-31.

AIDS patients are falling into the cracks of the insurance, social security, medicare and medicaid systems. Costs for treating a patient range in the hundreds of thousands of dollars. Insurance companies are afraid of receiving many large claims and the government systems require that a patient be below the poverty level. The government needs to step in to ensure that every patient receives adequate care.

The Patent Rights to the AIDS Virus

370. "AIDS: Sharing Out the Spoils." <u>New Scientist</u>, v. 108, October 10, 1985, p. 14.
   The patent dispute between French and American researchers is heating up. The immense amount of money involved may cause both sides to take actions that are not necessarily in the best interests of finding a cure for AIDS.

371. Beardsley, Tim. "French Virus in the Picture." <u>Nature</u>, v. 320, April 17, 1986, p. 563.
   Robert Gallo has announced that one of his first papers on the AIDS virus contained a mislabeled electron monograph. This error will give his group even less credibility in the patent fight over rights to discovery of the virus.

372. Beardsley, Tim. "Pasteur Sues Over Patent." <u>Nature</u>, v. 318, December 19, 1985, p. 595.
   The Pasteur Institute has sued the U.S. National Cancer Institute for patent infringements on the AIDS blood test. The French group was the first to identify the virus and file for a patent, but the patent was given to an American research team instead.

373. Carey, Joseph. "The Rivalry to Defeat AIDS." <u>U.S. News and World Report</u>, v. 100, January 13, 1986, pp. 67-68.
   American and French researchers are involved in a race to find a cure for AIDS. French scientists have sued the U.S. over priority rights in the discovery of the AIDS virus. The winning team will most likely win the Nobel Prize and receive millions of dollars in royalties.

374. Connor, Steve. "Americans Stop Talks About AIDS Discovery." <u>New Scientist</u>, v. 110, May 15, 1986, p. 30.
   Talks between American and French researchers over patent rights related to the AIDS virus have been broken off. The U.S. Patent Office has declared the French to be the senior party, but the Department of Human Services refuses to acknowledge that finding.

375. Gilbert, Susan. "The AIDS Controversies." <u>Science Digest</u>, v. 93, September 1985, p. 28.
   Competition and controversy have broken out between French and American scientists over the priority rights to the identification of the AIDS virus. American scientists may have misclassified AIDS as a retrovirus when it may actually be a lentivirus.

376. Gilden, Raymond V. et al. "HTLV-III Legend Correction." Science, v. 232, April 18, 1986, p. 307.

The electron micrograph appearing in the May 4, 1984 article in Science was mislabeled as an HTLV-III virus when in fact it was the LAV virus. This letter corrects that error.

377. "A Lawsuit on AIDS." Newsweek, v. 106, December 23, 1985, p. 65.

The French Pasteur Institute has sued the U.S. government over priority rights in the discovery of the AIDS virus.

378. Marx, Jean L. "AIDS Virus Has New Name--Perhaps." Science, v. 232, May 9, 1986, pp. 696-700.

A committee on nomenclature has recommended "Human Immunodeficiency Virus" as the official name of the AIDS virus. Unfortunately, the discoverers of the HTLV-III virus refuse to use this new name because it may influence the patent court to award the rights to the French group.

379. Marx, Jean. L. "A Virus By Any Other Name..." Science, v. 227, March 22, 1985, pp. 1449-1451.

Genetic comparisons have now indicated that the viruses that are linked to AIDS are all variants of the same virus, although they are not identical. A committee has been set up to determine an official name for the virus.

380. "New AIDS Viruses Spark More Rivalry." New Scientist, v. 110, April 3, 1986, p. 20.

Both French and American researchers claim to have discovered new viruses similar to the one that causes AIDS. Both of these viruses come from West Africa and may be the missing link relating the human and animal forms of the virus.

381. Norman, Colin. "AIDS Patent Negotiations Break Down." Science, v. 232, May 16, 1986, p. 819.

The U.S. Patent Office appears to favor the French team in the patent fight over the AIDS virus. The determination that favors the French group is that the Pasteur Institute has been declared the senior party in the infringence suit.

382. Norman, Colin. "AIDS Priority Fight Goes to Court." Science, v. 231, January 3, 1986, pp. 11-12.

The Pasteur Institute has filed suit against the National Institutes of Health over patent rights to the AIDS virus. The suit claims that the Pasteur Institute should have claim to all royalties resulting from an AIDS blood test. This suit may have the unfortunate result of inhibiting collaboration in the search for an AIDS vaccine.

383. Norman, Colin. "A New Twist in AIDS Patent Fight." Science, v. 232, April 18, 1986, pp. 308-309.

A correction to an article in Science in 1984 may affect the legal status of the AIDS virus. Because the American team mislabeled their electron micrographs as HTLV-III instead of LAV, the French team may be able to use this fact in their patent suit.

384. Norman, Colin. "Patent Dispute Divides AIDS Researchers." Science, v. 230, November 8, 1985, pp. 640-642.

Although a group headed by Robert Gallo published the first papers on the AIDS virus, the French research group that had first worked with the virus felt that they did not receive proper credit. The French group has filed a patent suit against the National Cancer Institute and a committee has been established to review the naming of the AIDS virus.

385. Palca, Joseph. "Controversy Over AIDS Virus Extends to Name." Nature, v. 321, May 1, 1986, p. 3.

A committee on nomenclature has recommended that Human Immunodeficiency Virus (HIV) become the standard name of the AIDS virus. Unfortunately, some of the key individuals involved in the naming controversy refuse to adopt the new name.

386. Palca, Joseph. "U.S. Plans for Foundation in Trouble with French." Nature, v. 321, May 15, 1986, p. 185.

The U.S. Department of Health and Human Services intends to establish an international foundation for research on AIDS. French researchers claim that this is a public relations ploy to prevent the French from receiving patent rights to the virus.

387. Rhein, Reginald. "A French Claim on AIDS Testing." Chemical Week, v. ???, October 16, 1985, p. 11.

The French researchers who initially filed for a patent on the AIDS virus are threatening to sue the U.S. government over rights to the AIDS blood test. Blood test kits should have an initial market of at least $80 million.

388. Sattaur, Omar. "How Gallo Got Credit for the AIDS Discovery." New Scientist, v. 105, February 7, 1985, pp. 3-4.

Growing evidence suggests that Robert Gallo has misclassified the AIDS virus and that the French researchers have found the real AIDS virus. Recent publications of the genetic code indicates that AIDS is caused by a retrovirus, not by an HTLV virus. Despite this evidence, Gallo is still being given credit for the discovery.

389. Walgate, Robert and Tim Beardsley. "Pasteur Plans to Pursue Suit on Virus." Nature, v. 320, March 13, 1986, p. 96.

The Pasteur Institute will continue its lawsuit against the National Institutes of Health over patent rights to the AIDS virus. New evidence indicates that the American researchers were able to propagate the LAV virus found by French scientists, which the Americans claim did not survive in their laboratory.

390. Walgate, Robert and Tim Beardsley. "U.S. and French Institutes in Patent Struggle." Nature, v. 317, October 3, 1985, p. 373.

The recent development of the AIDS blood test is causing a dispute between French and American scientists over patent rights. While the French researchers filed first, the patent was given to the American team. The Patent Office will issue a ruling in the future on who should be given priority rights for the AIDS virus.

391. "What's In a Name?" Nature, v. 321, May 1, 1986, p. 2.

The fight over rights to the AIDS virus is complicated by the many names for the virus. A committee has recommended the name Human Immunodeficiency Virus (HIV), but only time will tell if this will help solve the problem.

392. "Why the AIDS Virus Is Not Like HTLVs-I or -II." New Scientist, v. 105, February 7, 1986, p. 4.

The AIDS virus is not an HTLV, but a retrovirus. The genetic sequences of HTLV and LAV are compared.

Services for AIDS Victims

393. Chamberland, Mary E. et al. "Acquired Immunodeficiency Syndrome in New York City." JAMA: Journal of the American Medical Association, v. 254, July 19, 1985, pp. 383-387.
   Describes the activities of the New York City AIDS surveillance program. This program is effective and is sufficiently complete for accurate analysis of disease trends.

394. Goldsmith, Marsha F. "Many Groups Offer AIDS Information, Support." JAMA: Journal of the American Medical Association, v. 254, November 8, 1985, pp. 2522-2523.
   Many AIDS information centers have been established throughout the country. A directory of national, regional, and local centers is provided.

395. Goodman, Eric. "AIDS: Beneath the Sign of the Cross." Life, v. 9, February 1986, p. 27.
   Efforts to establish a hospice for children with AIDS in rural Virginia was met by anger from local residents. At a town meeting, the response was so negative that the hospice plan was terminated.

396. Helgerson, Steven D. "AIDS Project in Seattle, Washington." American Journal of Public Health, v. 74, December 1984, p. 1419.
   The Seattle city and county governments have established an AIDS assessment, education, and surveillance project. Activities include an AIDS hotline, publications, and an AIDS risk assessment clinic.

397. Leishman, Katie. "A Crisis in Public Health." Atlantic, v. 256, October 1985, pp. 18-41.
   San Francisco has done more to help AIDS patients than any other city in the world. The history of AIDS in San Francisco and the responses of the community and government are detailed.

398. Lopez, Diego J. and George S. Getzel. "Helping Gay AIDS Patients in Crisis." Social Casework, v. 65, September 1984, pp. 387-394.
   AIDS affects the gay community biologically, psychologically, and sociologically. The Gay Men's Health Crisis was founded to assist AIDS patients. The history of the organization and a case study of the support system in action are provided.

399. Morin, Stephen F. "AIDS in One City." American Psychologist, v. 39, November 1984, pp. 1294-1296.
   The city of San Francisco has responded to AIDS by establishing a number of services and programs for victims. Mervyn Silverman, city health director, describes how San Francisco is helping AIDS patients.

400. Morrisroe, Patricia. "The Guardian Angel." New York, v. 18, December 9, 1985, pp. 46-51.

The story of a man who provides personal home care for seriously ill AIDS patients. He has seen 27 patients die and worries about contracting the disease himself. However, he will continue to provide his unique services as long as possible.

Rock Hudson: AIDS Strikes a Star

401. Barber, John. "Rock Hudson and the War Against AIDS." <u>Macleans</u>, v. 98, August 5, 1985, p. 44.

Rock Hudson has announced that he is suffering from AIDS, making him the first celebrity to publicly disclose AIDS. Mr. Hudson has gone to Paris in hopes of finding help with an experimental treatment.

402. Barol, Bill. "A Hollywood Bash to Combat AIDS." <u>Newsweek</u>, v. 106, September 30, 1985, pp. 80-81.

A number of celebrities have worked together to put on a special show to raise funding for AIDS research in the memory of Rock Hudson.

403. Clarke, Gerald. "The Double Life of an AIDS Victim." <u>Time</u>, v. 126, October 14, 1985, p. 106.

The death of Rock Hudson temporarily made him the most famous homosexual man in the world, a fact that he had kept secret for 59 years. His life and the disease that led to his death are discussed.

404. Gelman, David and Michael Reese. "AIDS Strikes a Star." <u>Newsweek</u>, v. 106, August 5, 1985, pp. 68-69.

Rock Hudson has been admitted to a French hospital to try an experimental treatment for AIDS. The film community is very concerned about the health of one of its friends and the gay community feels that funding and research will be increased now that a "star" has contracted the disease.

405. Haller, Scot. "Fighting for Life." <u>People</u>, v. 24, September 23, 1985, pp. 28-33.

The motion picture and television industry is very concerned about AIDS, especially after the death of Rock Hudson. Many actors and actresses are quoted in their fight against the disease.

406. "Rock Hudson." <u>People</u>, v. 24, December 23, 1985, pp. 108-111.

Rock Hudson's admission of AIDS stunned the world and helped to spur contributions to AIDS research. Some actors are now afraid to kiss for fear of catching the disease and Rock Hudson's lover is suing the estate for damages due to failure to notify him about the disease.

407. "Rock Hudson AIDS Case Sends a Message." <u>U.S. News and World Report</u>, v. 99, August 5, 1985, p. 12.

Rock Hudson's admission that he has AIDS has brought a great deal of attention to the disease. He is currently in France seeking experimental treatments with the drug HPA-23.

408. Wallis, Claudia. "AIDS: A Spreading Scourge." <u>Time</u>, v. 126, August 5, 1985, pp. 50-51.

When AIDS struck Rock Hudson, the public became even more aware of the pervasiveness of the disease. It strikes people of all walks of life and no one has ever recovered. Researchers need more funding and direction if they are to find a cure.

409. Yarbrough, J. "Rock Hudson: On Camera and Off." <u>People</u>, v. 24, August 12, 1985, pp. 34-41.

A biography of Rock Hudson from his childhood through his acting career and his death due to AIDS.

AIDS Outside the United States

410. "Africa's Latest Torment: AIDS." <u>U.S. News and World Report</u>, v. 99, December 23, 1985, p. 8.
    AIDS has been found in twenty-five central African nations. Hundreds of thousands of victims may have the disease, which affects both men and women equally. African governments are trying to cover up their AIDS problems to avoid negative publicity.

411. "AIDS Cases Reported in European Centre." <u>World Health</u>, December 1985, pp. 30-31.
    Eighteen European countries have reported cases of AIDS and the rate is increasing at twenty-two per week. The demographics and epidemiology of AIDS in Europe are described.

412. "AIDS in a Heterosexual Population." <u>American Family Physician</u>, v. 31, February 1985, p. 292.
    AIDS in Africa has a one-to-one male to female ratio and is not linked to homosexuality, drug abuse, hemophilia, or blood transfusions. This provides strong evidence of heterosexual transmission of the virus.

413. "AIDS in Africa." <u>New Scientist</u>, v. 108, November 28, 1985, p. 14.
    African governments are not enthusiastic about the idea that AIDS originated in central Africa. This political problem must be solved so that a cure for the disease can be found.

414. "AIDS in Arabia." <u>New Scientist</u>, v. 109, January 30, 1986, p. 23.
    While only three cases of AIDS have been found in the Arab world, Kuwait, Saudi Arabia, and the United Arab Emirates have begun testing of all blood donors. Anyone from another nation applying for work in those countries may also be tested.

415. Clarke, Maxine. "New Cases Cause Alarm." <u>Nature</u>, v. 314, March 7, 1985, p. 5.
    Since the summer of 1982, 132 cases of AIDS have been reported in Britain, with 58 fatalities so far. British government policies and funding levels related to AIDS are presented.

416. Davis, Lisa. "AIDS: New Virus to Fill in the Blanks." <u>Science News</u>, v. 129, April 5, 1986, p. 212.
    Two new AIDS viruses have recently been discovered in West Africa. These may be the missing links between the human and animal viruses.

417. "Investigation Begins Into Spread of New AIDS Virus." *New Scientist*, v. 110, April 10, 1986, p. 25.

French researchers are trying to determine the extent of infection from a newly discovered African AIDS virus.

418. Harfi, Harb A. and Benyamin M. Fakhry. "Acquired Immunodeficiency Syndrome in Saudi Arabia." *JAMA: Journal of the American Medical Association*, v. 255, January 17, 1986, pp. 383-384.

One Saudi adult and one Saudi child developed AIDS 2.5 and 3.5 years after receiving blood transfusions. These are the first reported cases in Saudi Arabia. The blood used had been imported from the United States. Measures must be taken to prevent the importation of contaminated blood supplies.

419. Jayaraman, K. S. "India Against AIDS." *Nature*, v. 318, November 21, 1985, p. 201.

AIDS has not been found in India or Bangladesh, but a confirmed case in Pakistan is causing both countries to undertake an educational program and plan for an AIDS prevention program.

420. Johnstone, Bob. "Japan Blames U.S. Blood for AIDS Cases." *New Scientist*, v. 106, July 4, 1985, p. 22.

Five cases of AIDS have been detected in Japan. It is theorized that blood imported from the United States contained the AIDS virus.

421. Newmark, Peter. "Trailing AIDS in Central Africa." *Nature*, v. 315, May 23, 1985, p. 273.

AIDS seems to have originated in central Africa, possibly in Zaire. The issue is complicated by possible mutations in the virus and the insensitivity of AIDS tests. It now appears that the virus originated with the African Green Monkey.

422. Norman, Colin. "Africa and the Origin of AIDS." *Science*, v. 230, December 6, 1985, p. 1141.

AIDS appears to have originated in Africa, where it began as a mutated virus found in Green Monkeys. The African strains of the AIDS virus also appear to be more closely related to the animal version than strains from other parts of the world. African scientists and governments do not want that continent to be blamed for originating AIDS.

423. Norman, Colin. "Politics and Science Clash on African AIDS." *Science*, v. 230, December 6, 1985, pp. 1140-1142.

While African governments have not reported any cases of AIDS in central Africa, scientists have found that the disease is reaching alarming proportions. This political censorship is complicating the study of AIDS on that continent. The African version of the disease is present in equal numbers in men and women and is not limited to any high-risk groups.

424. "Prevalence of HTLV-III Infection in London." <u>American Family Physician</u>, v. 33, February 1986, p. 306.

A British study measured the presence of antibodies to the AIDS virus in blood samples taken in 1982 and 1984. The rate increased from 6.5% in 1982 to 21.6% in 1984. This follows the same rate of increase that was seen in San Francisco a few years ago.

425. Rich, Vera. "Poland's Minister for Prophylaxis." <u>Nature</u>, v. 317, September 12, 1985, p. 100.

The Polish government has appointed a special minister to study the AIDS crisis. AIDS has become a problem in Poland because a poor pharmaceutical industry has forced health care facilities to reuse needles and other equipment and drug addiction is on the increase. A mass screening of blood donors is being planned.

426. Rich, Vera. "Soviet Offer on AIDS." <u>Nature</u>, v. 317, October 24, 1985, p. 659.

While Soviet doctors will not admit that AIDS has been reported in that nation, they are offering to work with American physicians in the fight against the disease.

427. Rich, Vera. "Soviets Admit AIDS Cases." <u>Nature</u>, v. 318, December 12, 1985, p. 502.

A Soviet doctor has admitted that AIDS exists in the Soviet Union. This is contrary to the denial of its existence by other Soviet officials.

428. Sattaur, Omar. "African AIDS Points to Heterosexual Link." <u>New Scientist</u>, v. 106, April 25, 1985, pp. 10-11.

Studies in Zaire indicate that AIDS is transmitted through heterosexual contact and that many more people are at risk than previously thought. The evidence linking AIDS to heterosexual transmission is that the ratio of men to women with AIDS in Africa is one to one, there is a wide range of other sexually transmitted diseases in the same population, there are distinct clusters of AIDS victims, and 75% of spouses of victims have antibodies to the virus.

429. Sattaur, Omar. "Scientists Attack AIDS Slur on Africa." <u>New Scientist</u>, v. 108, November 28, 1985, pp. 15-16.

African scientists view the claim that the AIDS virus originated on that continent as a slur against Africa. This theory is still the source of controversy, but it appears that the AIDS virus is a mutated form of a similar virus often found in African Green Monkeys.

430. "Update: Acquired Immunodeficiency Syndrome: Europe." Updated regularly in MMWR: Morbidity and Mortality Weekly Report.

A regular feature of the MMWR that reports on cases of AIDS in Europe and in other regions of the world, including Africa and the Caribbean.

Animal AIDS

431. Kanki, Phyllis J. et al. "New Human T-Lymphotropic Retrovirus Related to Simian T-Lymphotropic Virus Type III (STLV-III$_{agm}$)." Science, v. 232, April 11, 1986, pp. 238-243.

A new virus similar to the simian HTLV-III virus has been found in humans in Senegal, West Africa. This virus will help in the study of AIDS and may be a link between the human and animal versions.

432. Kanki, Phyllis J. et al. "Serologic Identification and Characterization of a Macaque T-Lymphotropic Retrovirus Closely Related to HTLV-III." Science, v. 228, June 7, 1985, pp. 1199-1201.

A new virus similar to HTLV-III has been isolated in Macaque monkeys. This new virus, named STLV-III, may be useful in studying the human virus and the pathogenesis of AIDS.

433. Letvin, N. L. et al. "Induction of AIDS-Like Disease in Macaque Monkeys with T-Cell Tropic Retrovirus STLV-III." Science, v. 230, October 4, 1985, pp. 71-73.

Six rhesus monkeys were injected with the AIDS virus and four died of the disease within 160 days. This indicates that animal AIDS can be a useful model for the study of human AIDS.

434. Marx, Jean L. "New Relatives of AIDS Virus Found." Science, v. 232, April 11, 1986, p. 157.

Two new varieties of the AIDS virus have been discovered in West Africa and may be the link between the animal and human forms of the disease.

435. Silberner, J. "The AIDS Virus: Equine Similarities?" Science News, v. 129, February 8, 1986, p. 84.

The AIDS virus is similar to a virus that causes an infectious, sometimes fatal disease in horses. While this may make it easier to study the effects of the AIDS virus, it may also mean that it will be more difficult to develop a vaccine.

Author Index

Name: Abstract Number(s).

Abrams, D. I.: 1, 277, 301.
Abramson, P.: 91.
Adler, J.: 216, 281.
Agrest, S.: 246.
Allan, G.: 260.
Allan, J. S.: 5.
Allen, G.: 219, 220.
Allen, J. S.: 136.
Alter, J.: 221.
Amiel, B.: 222.
Anderson, I.: 165.
Barber, J.: 84, 224, 401.
Barin, F.: 6.
Barnes, F.: 225.
Barol, B.: 402.
Barre-Sinoussi, F.: 7.
Batchelor, W. F.: 302, 303, 313.
Baum, R.: 8.
Bayer, R.: 106, 226.
Beardsley, T.: 85, 166, 167, 284, 351, 352, 371, 372, 389, 390.
Beauchamp, M.: 168.
Bennett, D. D.: 304.
Bennett, J. A.: 49.
Black, D.: 227.
Blackwell, M.: 261.
Blaun, R.: 169.
Brandt, E. N.: 353.
Breu, G.: 143.
Bruno, M.: 320.
Buckley, W. F.: 228.
Budiansky, S.: 86, 87, 354.
Burda, D.: 355.
Burkes, R. L.: 9.
Bush, L.: 366.
Caputo, L.: 134.
Carey, J.: 373.
Carlson, J. R.: 88.
Carlson, P.: 262.
Castro, K. G.: 50.
Cecchi, R.: 229.
Chamberland, M. E.: 393.
Chang, N. T.: 89.
Charles, K. A.: 314.
Check, W.: 230.

Church, G. J.: 51.
Clark, M.: 91, 170-172.
Clarke, G.: 321, 403.
Clarke, M.: 92, 93, 415.
Coates, T. J.: 305, 326.
Conant, J.: 144, 339.
Connor, S.: 94, 374.
Cornish, E.: 322.
Crovella, A. C.: 263.
Curran, J. W.: 50, 52, 64, 95.
Dalton, S.: 23.
Davis, J.: 173.
Davis, L.: 174, 416.
Dilley, J. W.: 307.
Drotman, D. P.: 64.
Echenberg, D. F.: 145.
Eckert, R. D.: 96.
Fakhry, B. M.: 418.
Ferrara, A. J.: 264.
Fierman, J.: 97.
Finlayson, A.: 98.
Firshein, J.: 298.
Francis, D. P.: 177.
Franklin, D.: 232.
Gauthier, M.: 53.
Gelman, D.: 323, 404.
Gergen, D. R.: 233.
Gest, T.: 332.
Getzel, G. S.: 398.
Gilbert, S.: 375.
Gilden, R.: 376.
Ginzburg, H. M.: 105, 135.
Glasbrenner, K.: 285.
Goedert, J. J.: 54.
Goldsmith, M. F.: 99, 146, 178, 234, 394.
Goodman, E.: 395.
Gottlieb, M. S.: 12.
Greenberg, N. F.: 269, 281.
Greene, J.: 265.
Groocock, V.: 147.
Halcrow, A.: 287.
Haller, S.: 179, 266, 405.
Hammett, T. M.: 288, 289.
Hardy, A. M.: 50, 55, 136, 356.
Harfi, H. A.: 418.
Harrison, B. G.: 235.
Helgerson, S. D.: 396.
Heneson, N.: 180, 181, 236.
Holden, C.: 357.

Horstman, W.: 326.
Hyatt, J.: 333.
Jason, J.: 103.
Jayaraman, K. S.: 151, 419.
Johnstone, B.: 15, 104, 420.
Joseph, J. G.: 308.
Joyce, C.: 181.
Kanki, P. J.: 431, 432.
Kaplan, J. E.: 56.
Kenton, C.: 16.
King, S. H.: 358.
Klass, P.: 238.
Klatzmann, D.: 184.
Kocolowski, L.: 292.
Koplan, J. P.: 136.
Krause, R. M.: 185.
Kristal, A. R.: 17.
Landesman, S. H.: 105.
Langone, J.: 18, 186.
Lashley, T.: 298.
Laurence, J.: 19.
Leishman, K.: 397.
Letvin, N. L.: 433.
Levin, B.: 324.
Levine, C.: 106.
Linke, R. A.: 23.
Lonberg, M.: 22.
Lopez, D. J.: 398.
Lundberg, G. D.: 325.
Lunsden, A.: 239.
Maddox, J.: 309.
Malyon, A. K.: 314.
Mandel, J.: 305.
Mano, D. K.: 240.
Martin, J. L.: 310.
Martin, T.: 152.
Marwick, C.: 20, 107, 198, 241, 311.
Marx, J. L.: 57, 187, 188, 378, 379, 434.
Mason, J. O.: 21, 293.
Mayer, K. H.: 58.
McCoy, K.: 153.
McDonald, M.: 108.
McGrath, E.: 342.
McKusick, L.: 326, 327.
Meer, J.: 312.
Meldrum, J.: 59.
Miller, P. J.: 334.
Miller, R. W.: 109.
Montagnier, L.: 184.

Morin, S. F.: 313, 314, 399.
Morrisroe, P.: 267, 400.
Morrow, L.: 242.
Muggia, F. M.: 22.
Newmark, P.: 421.
Nieckarz, J.: 347.
Norman, C.: 61, 62, 111, 191, 192, 294, 360-363, 381-384, 422, 423.
Norman, M.: 315.
Norwood, C.: 154.
Ohlendorf, P.: 193, 194.
O'Sullivan, P.: 23.
Pahwa, S.: 155.
Palca, J.: 385, 386.
Panem, S.: 365.
Patton, C.: 262.
Pave, I.: 295.
Peabody, B.: 268.
Pedersen, D.: 246.
Perry, S. W.: 316.
Peterman, T. A.: 64, 112.
Peterson, F.: 113.
Petricciani, J. C.: 177.
Pincus, H. A.: 137.
Powills, S.: 355.
Press, A.: 246, 335.
Prout, L. R.: 144.
Quinn, T. C.: 26.
Ratner, L.: 28.
Redfield, R. R.: 158.
Reed, S.: 344.
Reese, M.: 404.
Relman, A. S.: 247.
Rhein, R.: 387.
Rich, V.: 425-427.
Riesenberg, D. E.: 198, 328.
Rock, A.: 116.
Rodman, T. C.: 30.
Sattaur, O.: 31, 117-119, 159, 317, 348, 388, 428, 429.
Schulte, L.: 329.
Scott, G. B.: 160.
Seale, J.: 32.
Seligmann, J.: 270, 331.
Serrill, M. S.: 248.
Servaas, C.: 68.
Shahoda, T.: 298.
Shaw, G. M.: 318.
Shelp, E. E.: 349.
Shine, D.: 138.
Silberner, J.: 69-71, 120, 121, 161, 199-203, 435.

Silverman, D. B.: 250.
Silverman, M. F.: 250.
Siwolop, S.: 204.
Sobran, J.: 251.
Spechko, P. L.: 271.
Spencer, N.: 122.
Stein, M. L.: 254.
Stevens, C. E.: 33.
Sullivan, M.: 289.
Sunderland, R. H.: 349.
Svesko, V.: 255.
Swinbanks, D.: 123, 124.
Switzer, E.: 162.
Talbot, D.: 366.
Tancredi, L. R.: 256.
Tanne, J. H.: 72.
Taravella, S.: 299.
Teitelman, R.: 125, 206.
Temshok, L.: 305.
Thomas, E.: 257.
Ticer, S.: 207.
Trafford, A.: 258.
Tross, S.: 316.
Vance, C. S.: 310.
Vaux, K.: 350.
Volberding, P. A.: 36, 277.
Volkow, N. D.: 256.
Wachter, R. M.: 278.
Waldman, S.: 369.
Walgate, R.: 37, 130, 209, 389, 390.
Wallis, C.: 77, 210, 408.
Weber, J.: 211.
Weiss, S. W.: 105, 131, 279.
White, E.: 227.
Wormser, G. P.: 39.
Wright, K.: 212, 213.
Yanchinski, S.: 132, 133.
Yarbrough, J.: 409.
Young, L. S.: 215.
Zimmerman, D. R.: 164.

LIBRARY USE ONLY
DOES NOT CIRCULATE